State of the Art Evaluation of the Head and Neck

Editor

ASHOK SRINIVASAN

NEUROIMAGING CLINICS OF NORTH AMERICA

www.neuroimaging.theclinics.com

Consulting Editor
SURESH K. MUKHERJI

August 2020 • Volume 30 • Number 3

ELSEVIER

1600 John F. Kennedy Boulevard • Suite 1800 • Philadelphia, Pennsylvania, 19103-2899

http://www.neuroimaging.theclinics.com

NEUROIMAGING CLINICS OF NORTH AMERICA Volume 30, Number 3
August 2020 ISSN 1052-5149, ISBN 13: 978-0-323-75588-7

Editor: John Vassallo (j.vassallo@elsevier.com)
Developmental Editor: Casey Potter

Neuroimaging Clinics of North America (ISSN 1052-5149) is published quarterly by Elsevier Inc., 360 Park Avenue South, New York, NY 10010-1710. Months of issue are February, May, August, and November. Business and editorial offices: 1600 John F. Kennedy Blvd., Suite 1800, Philadelphia, PA 19103-2899. Business and editorial offices: 6277 Sea Harbor Drive, Orlando, FL 32887-4800. Periodicals postage paid at New York, NY, and additional mailing offices. Subscription prices are USD 397 per year for US individuals, USD 686 per year for US institutions, USD 100 per year for US students and residents, USD 451 per year for Canadian individuals, USD 874 per year for Canadian institutions, USD 541 per year for international individuals, USD 874 per year for international institutions, USD 100 per year for Canadian students and residents and USD 260 per year for foreign students and residents. To receive student/resident rate, orders must be accompanied by name of affiliated institution, date of term, and the *signature* of program/residency coordinator on institution letterhead. Orders will be billed at individual rate until proof of status is received. Foreign air speed delivery is included in all *Clinics* subscription prices. All prices are subject to change without notice. POSTMASTER: Send address changes to *Neuroimaging Clinics of North America*, Elsevier Health Sciences Division, Subscription **Customer Service, 3251 Riverport Lane, Maryland Heights, MO 63043. Telephone: 1-800-654-2452 (U.S. and Canada); 314-447-8871 (outside U.S. and Canada). Fax: 314-447-8029. E-mail: journalscustomerservice-usa@elsevier.com (for print support); journalsonlinesupport-usa@elsevier.com (for online support).**

Reprints. For copies of 100 or more of articles in this publication, please contact the Commercial Reprints Department, Elsevier Inc., 360 Park Avenue South, New York, NY 10010-1710. Tel.: 212-633-3874; Fax: 212-633-3820; E-mail: reprints@elsevier.com.

Neuroimaging Clinics of North America is covered by *Excerpta Medical/EMBASE,* the RSNA Index of Imaging Literature, *MEDLINE/PubMed (Index Medicus),* MEDLINE/MEDLARS, SciSearch, Research Alert, and Neuroscience Citation Index.

PROGRAM OBJECTIVE

The goal of *Neuroimaging Clinics of North America* is to keep practicing radiologists and radiology residents up to date with current clinical practice in radiology by providing timely articles reviewing the state of the art in patient care.

TARGET AUDIENCE

Practicing radiologists, radiology residents, and other healthcare professionals who utilize neuroimaging findings to provide patient care.

LEARNING OBJECTIVES

Upon completion of this activity, participants will be able to:

1. Review recent updates on the latest tools in the imaging armamentarium for head and neck evaluation.
2. Discuss various imaging modalities and techniques such as diffusion imaging, MR spectroscopy, technological improvements in MRI, dual energy CT and PET-CT.
3. Recognize key features and categories to incorporate into standardizing the radiologist report and the potential impact on management of the patient.

ACCREDITATION

The Elsevier Office of Continuing Medical Education (EOCME) is accredited by the Accreditation Council for Continuing Medical Education (ACCME) to provide continuing medical education for physicians.

The EOCME designates this journal-based CME activity for a maximum of 9 *AMA PRA Category 1 Credit*(s)™. Physicians should claim only the credit commensurate with the extent of their participation in the activity.

All other healthcare professionals requesting continuing education credit for this enduring material will be issued a certificate of participation.

DISCLOSURE OF CONFLICTS OF INTEREST

The EOCME assesses conflict of interest with its instructors, faculty, planners, and other individuals who are in a position to control the content of CME activities. All relevant conflicts of interest that are identified are thoroughly vetted by EOCME for fair balance, scientific objectivity, and patient care recommendations. EOCME is committed to providing its learners with CME activities that promote improvements or quality in healthcare and not a specific proprietary business or a commercial interest.

The planning committee, staff, authors and editors listed below have identified no financial relationships or relationships to products or devices they or their spouse/life partner have with commercial interest related to the content of this CME activity:

Jay Acharya, MD; Mohit Agarwal, MD; Glenn D. Barest, MD; V. Carlota Andreu-Arasa, MD, PhD; Jeffrey Chankowsky, MD; Noriyuki Fujima, MD, PhD; Wende Gibbs, MD; John L. Go, MD, FACR; Derek Hsu, MD; Amy F. Juliano, MD; Marilu Kelly, MSN, RN, CNE, CHCP; Rihan Khan, MD; Paul E. Kim, MD; Nicholas A. Koontz, MD; Pradeep Kuttysankaran; Luke Ledbetter, MD; Chia-Shang J. Liu, MD, PhD; Farhad Maleki, PhD; Juan Camilo Marquez, MD; Suresh K. Mukherji, MD, MBA, FACR; Nikesh Muthukrishnan, MEng; Carrie D. Norris, MD; Jason G. Parker, PhD, BS; Vishal Patel, MD, PhD; Sandra E. Quick, MD; Anandh G. Rajamohan, MD; Osamu Sakai, MD, PhD, FACR; Thiparom Sananmuang, MD; Marc Seltzer, MD; Nasim Sheikh-Bahaei, MD, PhD; Monica Shukla, MD; Ashok Srinivasan, MD, DNB; John Vassallo; Kyle Werth, MD.

The planning committee, staff, authors and editors listed below have identified financial relationships or relationships to products or devices they or their spouse/life partner have with commercial interest related to the content of this CME activity:

Gregory Avey, MD: consultant/advisor for General Electric Company.

Reza Forghani, MD, PhD: speaker's bureau, consultant/advisor and research support from General Electric Company; stock ownership in 4intelligent Inc.

UNAPPROVED/OFF-LABEL USE DISCLOSURE

The EOCME requires CME faculty to disclose to the participants:

1. When products or procedures being discussed are off-label, unlabelled, experimental, and/or investigational (not US Food and Drug Administration [FDA] approved); and
2. Any limitations on the information presented, such as data that are preliminary or that represent ongoing research, interim analyses, and/or unsupported opinions. Faculty may discuss information about pharmaceutical agents that is outside of FDA-approved labelling. This information is intended solely for CME and is not intended to promote off-label use of these medications. If you have any questions, contact the medical affairs department of the manufacturer for the most recent prescribing information.

TO ENROLL

To enroll in the *Neuroimaging Clinics of North America* Continuing Medical Education program, call customer service at 1-800-654-2452 or sign up online at http://www.theclinics.com/home/cme. The CME program is available to subscribers for an additional annual fee of USD 245.00.

METHOD OF PARTICIPATION

In order to claim credit, participants must complete the following:

1. Complete enrolment as indicated above.
2. Read the activity.
3. Complete the CME Test and Evaluation. Participants must achieve a score of 70% on the test. All CME Tests and Evaluations must be completed online.

CME INQUIRIES/SPECIAL NEEDS

For all CME inquiries or special needs, please contact elsevierCME@elsevier.com.

NEUROIMAGING CLINICS OF NORTH AMERICA

SERIES OF RELATED INTEREST

Advances in Clinical Radiology
Advancesinclinicalradiology.com
MRI Clinics of North America
Mri.theclinics.com
PET Clinics
pet.theclinics.com
Radiologic Clinics of North America
Radiologic.theclinics.com

THE CLINICS ARE AVAILABLE ONLINE!
Access your subscription at:
www.theclinics.com

Contributors

CONSULTING EDITOR

SURESH K. MUKHERJI, MD, MBA, FACR
Clinical Professor, Marian University, Director
of Head and Neck Radiology, ProScan
Imaging, Regional Medical Director, Envision
Physician Services, Carmel, Indiana, USA

EDITOR

ASHOK SRINIVASAN, MD, DNB
Director of Neuroradiology, Michigan
Medicine, Professor of Radiology, University of
Michigan, Ann Arbor, Michigan, USA

AUTHORS

JAY ACHARYA, MD
Assistant Professor of Clinical Radiology,
Department of Radiology, Division of
Neuroradiology, University of Southern
California, Keck School of Medicine of USC,
Los Angeles, California, USA

MOHIT AGARWAL, MD
Department of Radiology, Section of
Neuroradiology, Froedtert and Medical College
of Wisconsin, Milwaukee, Wisconsin, USA

GREGORY AVEY, MD
Associate Professor, Radiology, University of
Wisconsin-Madison, Madison, Wisconsin, USA

GLENN D. BAREST, MD
Clinical Associate Professor, Department of
Radiology, Boston Medical Center, Boston
University School of Medicine, Boston,
Massachusetts, USA

V. CARLOTA ANDREU-ARASA, MD, PhD
Assistant Professor, Department of Radiology,
Boston Medical Center, Boston University
School of Medicine, Boston, Massachusetts,
USA

JEFFREY CHANKOWSKY, MD
Department of Radiology, McGill University,
Montreal, Quebec, Canada

REZA FORGHANI, MD, PhD
Director and Lead Investigator, Augmented
Intelligence & Precision Health Laboratory,
Department of Radiology, Research Institute of
the McGill University Health Centre,
Department of Radiology, McGill University,
Segal Cancer Centre, Lady Davis Institute for
Medical Research, Jewish General Hospital,
Gerald Bronfman Department of Oncology,
McGill University, Department of
Otolaryngology–Head and Neck Surgery,
Royal Victoria Hospital, McGill University
Health Centre, Montreal, Quebec, Canada

NORIYUKI FUJIMA, MD, PhD
Research Scholar, Department of Radiology,
Boston Medical Center, Boston University
School of Medicine, Boston, Massachusetts,
USA; Research Fellow, Research Center for
Cooperative Projects, Hokkaido University
Graduate School of Medicine, Sapporo,
Hokkaido, Japan

WENDE GIBBS, MD
Senior Associate Consultant, Department of
Radiology, Mayo Clinic School of Medicine,
Scottsdale, Arizona, USA

JOHN L. GO, MD, FACR
Assistant Professor of Clinical Radiology,
Department of Radiology, Division of
Neuroradiology, University of Southern
California, Keck School of Medicine of USC,
Los Angeles, California, USA

DEREK HSU, MD
Department of Radiology and Imaging
Sciences, Emory School of Medicine, Atlanta,
Georgia, USA

AMY F. JULIANO, MD
Assistant Professor, Department of Radiology,
Massachusetts Eye and Ear, Harvard Medical
School, Boston, Massachusetts, USA

RIHAN KHAN, MD
Associate Professor, Department of Radiology,
Dartmouth-Hitchcock Medical Center,
Lebanon, New Hampshire, USA

PAUL E. KIM, MD
Associate Professor of Clinical Radiology,
Department of Radiology, Division of
Neuroradiology, University of Southern
California, Keck School of Medicine of USC,
Los Angeles, California, USA

NICHOLAS A. KOONTZ, MD
Director of Fellowship Programs, Dean D.T.
Maglinte Scholar in Radiology Education,
Assistant Professor, Departments of Radiology
and Imaging Sciences, and Otolaryngology–
Head and Neck Surgery, Indiana
University School of Medicine, Indianapolis,
Indiana, USA

LUKE LEDBETTER, MD
Department of Radiology, David Geffen School
of Medicine at UCLA, Los Angeles, California,
USA

CHIA-SHANG J. LIU, MD, PhD
Assistant Professor of Clinical Radiology,
Department of Radiology, Division of
Neuroradiology, University of Southern
California, Keck School of Medicine of USC,
Los Angeles, California, USA

FARHAD MALEKI, PhD
Augmented Intelligence & Precision Health
Laboratory, Department of Radiology.
Research Institute of the McGill University
Health Centre, Montreal, Quebec, Canada

JUAN CAMILO MARQUEZ, MD
Augmented Intelligence & Precision Health
Laboratory, Department of Radiology,
Research Institute of the McGill University
Health Centre, Department of Radiology,
McGill University, Montreal, Quebec, Canada

NIKESH MUTHUKRISHNAN, MEng
Augmented Intelligence & Precision Health
Laboratory, Department of Radiology,
Research Institute of the McGill University
Health Centre, Montreal, Quebec, Canada

CARRIE D. NORRIS, MD
Diagnostic Radiology Resident, Department of
Radiology and Imaging Sciences, Indiana
University School of Medicine, Indianapolis,
Indiana, USA

JASON G. PARKER, PhD, BS
Associate Professor, Department of Radiology
and Imaging Sciences, Indiana University
School of Medicine, Indianapolis, Indiana, USA

VISHAL PATEL, MD, PhD
Assistant Professor, Department of Radiology,
Division of Neuroradiology, USC Mark and
Mary Stevens Neuroimaging and Informatics
Institute, University of Southern California,
Keck School of Medicine of USC, Los Angeles,
California, USA

SANDRA E. QUICK, MD
Staff Neuroradiologist, Department of
Radiology, Richard L. Roudebush VA Medical
Center, Indianapolis, Indiana, USA

ANANDH G. RAJAMOHAN, MD
Assistant Professor of Clinical Radiology,
Department of Radiology, Division of
Neuroradiology, University of Southern
California, Keck School of Medicine of USC,
Los Angeles, California, USA

OSAMU SAKAI, MD, PhD, FACR
Chief of Neuroradiology, Professor of
Radiology, Otolaryngology–Head and Neck
Surgery, and Radiation Oncology, Boston

Medical Center, Boston University School of
Medicine, Boston, Massachusetts, USA

THIPAROM SANANMUANG, MD
Augmented Intelligence & Precision Health
Laboratory, Department of Radiology,
Research Institute of the McGill University
Health Centre, Montreal, Quebec, Canada;
Department of Diagnostic and Therapeutic
Radiology and Research, Faculty of Medicine,
Ramathibodi Hospital, Bangkok, Thailand

MARC SELTZER, MD
Professor, Department of Radiology,
Dartmouth-Hitchcock Medical Center,
Lebanon, New Hampshire, USA

NASIM SHEIKH-BAHAEI, MD, PhD
Assistant Professor of Clinical Radiology,
Department of Radiology, Division of

Neuroradiology, University of Southern
California, Keck School of Medicine of
USC, Los Angeles, California,
USA

MONICA SHUKLA, MD
Department of Radiation Oncology, Froedtert
and Medical College of Wisconsin, Milwaukee,
Wisconsin, USA

ASHOK SRINIVASAN, MD, DNB
Director of Neuroradiology, Michigan
Medicine, Professor of Radiology, University
of Michigan, Ann Arbor, Michigan,
USA

KYLE WERTH, MD
Department of Radiology, University of
Kansas Medical Center, Kansas City, Kansas,
USA

Contents

Diffusion imaging is a functional MR imaging tool that creates tissue contrast representative of the random, microscopic translational motion of water molecules within human body tissues. Long considered a cornerstone MR imaging sequence for brain imaging, diffusion-weighted imaging (DWI) increasingly is used for head and neck imaging. This review reports the current state of diffusion techniques for head and neck imaging, including conventional DWI, DWI trace with apparent diffusion coefficient map, diffusion tensor imaging, intravoxel incoherent motion, and diffusion kurtosis imaging. This article describes background physics, reports supportive evidence and potential pitfalls, highlights technical advances, and details practical clinical applications.

Several investigations have revealed the utility of magnetic resonance spectroscopy (MRS) as an adjunct in the evaluation of lesions of the head and neck. This technique remains a challenge in the head and neck because of its low signal-to-noise ratio and long acquisition times. In this review article, the basics of image acquisition technique and reported clinical utilities of head and neck MRS are presented.

Head and neck MR imaging is technically challenging because of magnetic field inhomogeneity, respiratory and swallowing motion, and necessity of high-resolution imaging to trace key anatomic structures. These challenges have been answered by advances in MR imaging technology, including isovolumetric three-dimensional imaging, robust fat-water separation techniques, and novel deep learning–based reconstruction algorithms. New applications of MR imaging have been advanced and functional imaging has been improved. Improvements in acquisition and reconstruction technique facilitate novel applications of morphologic and functional imaging. This results in opportunities to improve diagnosis, staging, and treatment selection through application of advanced MR imaging techniques.

> Multiple applications of dual energy computed tomography (DECT) have been described for the evaluation of disorders in the head and neck, especially in oncology. We review the body of evidence suggesting advantages of DECT for the evaluation of the neck compared with conventional single energy computed tomography scans, but the full potential of DECT is still to be realized. There is early evidence suggesting significant advantages of DECT for the extraction of quantitative biomarkers using radiomics and machine learning, representing a new horizon that may enable this technology to reach its full potential.

> Tumor hypoxia is a known independent prognostic factor for adverse patient outcomes in those with head and neck cancer. Areas of tumor hypoxia have been found to be more radiation resistant than areas of tumor with normal oxygenation levels. Hypoxia imaging may serve to help identify the best initial treatment option and to assess intratreatment monitoring of tumor response in case treatment changes can be made. PET imaging is the gold standard method for imaging tumor hypoxia, with 18F-fluoromisonidazole the most extensively studied hypoxic imaging tracer. Newer tracers also show promise.

> The traditional 'one-size-fits-all' approach to H&N cancer therapy is archaic. Advanced imaging can identify radioresistant areas by using biomarkers that detect tumor hypoxia, hypercellularity etc. Highly conformal radiotherapy can target resistant areas with precision. The critical information that can be gleaned about tumor biology from these advanced imaging modalities facilitates individualized radiotherapy. The tumor imaging world is pushing its boundaries. Molecular imaging can now detect protein expression and genotypic variations across tumors that can be exploited for tailoring treatment. The exploding field of radiomics and radiogenomics extracts quantitative, biologic and genetic information and further expands the scope of personalized therapy.

> Artificial intelligence, specifically machine learning and deep learning, is a rapidly developing field in imaging sciences with the potential to improve the efficiency and effectiveness of radiologists. This review covers common technical terms and basic concepts in imaging artificial intelligence and briefly reviews the application of these techniques to general imaging as well as head and neck imaging. Artificial intelligence has the potential to contribute improvements to all areas of patient care, including image acquisition, processing, segmentation, automated detection of findings, integration of clinical information, quality improvement, and research. Numerous challenges remain, however, before widespread imaging clinical adoption and integration occur.

Derek Hsu and Amy F. Juliano

Head and neck cancer surveillance imaging is diagnostically challenging, often with highly distorted anatomy after surgery and chemoradiation therapy. In the era of standardized reporting, the Neck Imaging Reporting and Data System (NI-RADS) was developed as a numerical classification system to provide clear and concise radiology reports and recommend next management step. There are 5 categories, each conveying a certain level of suspicion for the presence of persistent or recurrent disease. This article reviews the goals of NI-RADS, NI-RADS categories and lexicon, current research, and the future direction of NI-RADS in posttreatment head and neck cancer surveillance.

Anandh G. Rajamohan, Vishal Patel, Nasim Sheikh-Bahaei, Chia-Shang J. Liu, John L. Go, Paul E. Kim, Wende Gibbs, and Jay Acharya

Radiologists must convert the complex information in head and neck imaging into text reports that can be understood and used by clinicians, patients, and fellow radiologists for patient care, research, and quality initiatives. Common data elements in reporting, through use of defined questions with constrained answers and terminology, allow radiologists to incorporate best practice standards and improve communication of information regardless of individual reporting style. Use of common data elements for head and neck reporting has the potential to improve outcomes, reduce errors, and transition data consumption not only for humans but future machine learning systems.

Foreword

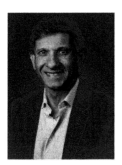

Suresh K. Mukherji, MD, MBA, FACR
Consulting Editor

This issue of *Neuroimaging Clinics*, entitled "State of the Art Evaluation of the Head and Neck," is devoted advanced techniques in head and neck imaging... a topic near and dear to my heart! This issue has articles specifically dedicated to head and neck applications of diffusion imaging, MR spectroscopy, technological improvements in MR imaging, dual-energy computed tomography (CT), PET-CT, and artificial intelligence post-treatment imaging.

I want to thank Ashok Srinivasan for accepting our invitation to guest edit this very important issue. I recruited Dr Srinivasan to the University of Michigan early in his career, and it has been a pleasure watching him and his equally talented wife (!) blossom into superb academic radiologists.

I would also like to personally thank all of the article authors. All contributors are both leaders in the field and recognized domain experts for their chosen topics. This wonderful issue would not be possible without your efforts, and all of us at *Neuroimaging Clinics* greatly appreciate your efforts. Your continued pursuit of new and innovative techniques will result in better outcomes for our patients. Thank you for helping to create the future of this wonderful and important specialty!

Suresh K. Mukherji, MD, MBA, FACR
Clinical Professor, Marian University
Director of Head and Neck Radiology
ProScan Imaging, Regional Medical Director
Envision Physician Services
Carmel, IN, USA

E-mail address:
sureshmukherji@hotmail.com

https://doi.org/10.1016/j.nic.2020.05.005
1052-5149/20/

Preface

Head and Neck Imaging in the Twenty-First Century

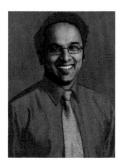

Ashok Srinivasan, MD, DNB
Editor

It is my honor and pleasure to put together this issue on "State of the Art Evaluation of the Head and Neck." I would like to thank the Consulting Editor, Dr Mukherji, for inviting me to guest edit this issue, and the publishers, for all their efforts at bringing this to fruition. I would also like to thank all the authors who have contributed superlative articles for inclusion in this issue. Truly speaking, this issue would not be possible without the dedication of all the authors, who have spent hours of their precious time creating high-quality educational articles.

Imaging evaluation of the head and neck can be a daunting task even for the experienced radiologist, especially due to the presence of complex fascial planes and the architectural distortion that results from surgical intervention and radiation therapy. The goal of this issue is to provide a comprehensive update on the latest tools in the imaging armamentarium for head and neck evaluation. Optimal deployment and utilization of these tools can help all radiologists navigate the landscape in both the pretreatment and posttreatment neck and provide a more meaningful evaluation.

A number of imaging modalities and techniques are discussed in detail in this issue. These include diffusion imaging, MR spectroscopy, technological improvements in MR imaging, dual-energy computed tomography (CT), and PET-CT. As we move into the next decade, it becomes more imperative to continue to establish value for novel imaging tools, incorporate them into standard-of-care imaging protocols, and provide the maximal benefit for our patients. There are also articles focused on the role of advanced imaging after radiation therapy, and the evolving landscape of artificial intelligence in head and neck imaging. The authors of all these articles have done a terrific job of breaking down the basics and emphasizing the clinical implications.

Last but not the least are articles focused on standardizing the most important end product of the radiologist: the dictated report. In the article on NI-RADS, the authors introduce the concept of providing clear categories of suspicion in posttreatment neck imaging and discuss how it can impact the management of the patient. In the article on common data elements, the authors stress the importance of using these elements in reports, and showcase different scenarios in head and neck imaging where these can be incorporated.

I enjoyed putting this issue together and hope that the readers get to benefit from the expertise of all the authors, who have contributed state-of-the-art articles.

Ashok Srinivasan, MD, DNB
Michigan Medicine
Department of Radiology, B2-A209D
University of Michigan
1500 East Medical Center Drive
Ann Arbor, MI 48109, USA

E-mail address:
ashoks@med.umich.edu

neuroimaging.theclinics.com

Neuroimag Clin N Am 30 (2020) xvii
https://doi.org/10.1016/j.nic.2020.05.004
1052-5149/20/© 2020 Published by Elsevier Inc.

Diffusion MR Imaging in the Head and Neck
Principles and Applications

Carrie D. Norris, MD[a], Sandra E. Quick, MD[b], Jason G. Parker, PhD, BS[a],
Nicholas A. Koontz, MD[a,c,*]

KEYWORDS

- Diffusion-weighted imaging (DWI) • Diffusion tensor imaging (DTI)
- Intravoxel incoherent motion (IVIM) • Diffusion kurtosis imaging (DKI) • Head and neck imaging
- MR imaging • Oncologic imaging • Cholesteatoma

KEY POINTS

- Diffusion imaging creates tissue contrast that reflects the random, microscopic translational motion of water molecules in the human body.
- Malignant tumors usually demonstrate lower mean apparent diffusion coefficient (ADC) values than benign tumors due to increased cellularity or high nuclear-to-cytoplasmic ratio. Remember, exceptions apply!
- Diffusion sequences should be viewed as complementary to routine MR imaging sequences, not as a replacement. Caution using mean ADC thresholds alone for predicting malignancy!
- Diffusion imaging improves sensitivity and specificity for detecting certain head and neck lesions, such as cholesteatoma, epidermoid cyst, abscess, and marrow replacement.
- Although some diffusion imaging techniques remain largely investigative, a growing body of evidence supports the routine use of diffusion imaging in the head and neck.

INTRODUCTION

Diffusion-weighted imaging (DWI) has long been considered a workhorse MR imaging pulse sequence for neuroimaging, particularly in the realm of stroke imaging. Over the past decade, DWI increasingly has become used for head and neck imaging applications, yet it remains an imperfect tool that can add value in many instances but generate confusion in others. Prone to certain artifacts (eg, geometric distortion, ghosting, magnetic susceptibility, incomplete fat saturation, and motion) and possessing relatively lower spatial resolution than conventional T1-weighted and T2-weighted sequences, precise anatomic localization of pathology on DWI sometimes is challenging[1,2] (Box 1). These shortcomings have left many radiologists with the impression that routine DWI in the head and neck is "not quite ready for prime time."

This review reports the current state of DWI in head and neck imaging, detailing salient background MR physics, potential pitfalls, supportive evidence, recent technical advances, and practical clinical applications (life hacks) that make DWI a prime time diagnostic tool in routine head and neck imaging.

[a] Department of Radiology and Imaging Sciences, Indiana University School of Medicine, 550 North University Boulevard, Room 0663, Indianapolis, IN 46202, USA; [b] Department of Radiology, Richard L. Roudebush VA Medical Center, 1481 West 10th Street, Indianapolis, IN 46202, USA; [c] Department of Otolaryngology–Head and Neck Surgery, Indiana University School of Medicine, Indianapolis, IN, USA
* Corresponding author. Department of Radiology and Imaging Sciences, 550 North University Boulevard, Room 0663, Indianapolis, IN 46202.
E-mail address: nakoontz@iupui.edu
Twitter: @CarrieDNorrisMD (C.D.N.); @nakoontz (N.A.K.)

PRINCIPLES OF DIFFUSION-WEIGHTED IMAGING

Diffusion MR imaging is a functional imaging modality that creates tissue contrast that is reflective of the random, microscopic translational motion of water molecules in the body. The rate of molecular motion in a homogenous fluid is driven by the size (mass) of the molecules and the presence of thermal energy and is defined by the Stokes-Einstein equation describing brownian motion.[3] In a homogeneous system, movement of water molecules is random and equal in all directions, thus characterized as isotropic. The human body is a highly heterogeneous system, however, with normal biologic systems and structures preventing water molecules from achieving true brownian motion. Instead, the translational motion of water molecules is impeded by structural elements (eg, axons or cytoskeleton) that exert

a preferential directionality to molecular movement, a feature called anisotropy. This feature can be exploited to gain insight into the molecular structure of tissue with advanced techniques, such as diffusion tensor imaging (DTI) and diffusion kurtosis imaging (DKI).

In certain pathologic states, the diffusivity of water molecules is reduced. In ischemic stroke, for example, brain cells are deprived of blood flow, thus starved of glucose substrates required to drive the adenosine triphosphate–dependent sodium-potassium pumps. This causes influx and sequestration of intracellular ions, which trap water molecules within the intracellular space via concentration gradients, leading to increased cellular size (ie, cellular swelling). The corresponding reduction in diffusivity of water molecules serves as the MR imaging surrogate for cytotoxic edema. In some tumors, free diffusivity of water molecules is impaired by the high cellularity or high nuclear-to-cytoplasmic ratio; thus, reduced diffusivity also is a surrogate marker for increased tumor cellularity (**Fig. 1**). Rooted in these basic concepts, diffusion imaging offers radiologists tools to identify infection/inflammation, improves detection of neoplasia, characterizes the biology of tumors, and monitors treatment response.[4,5]

DIFFUSION IMAGING VARIANTS
Conventional Diffusion-Weighted Imaging

In the simplest form of DWI, a single-pulsed echo planar sequence is acquired in 1 gradient direction. Acquisition time is short, can be effectively

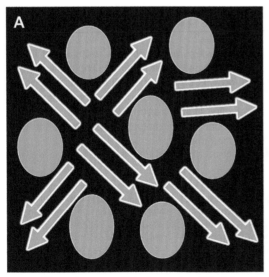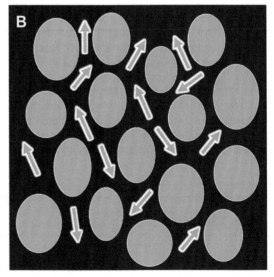

Fig. 1. Effect of tumor cellularity on the diffusivity of water molecules. Low-cellularity tumor (*A*) shows relatively high diffusivity of water molecules (*arrow vectors*), whereas high-cellularity tumor (*B*) shows reduced diffusivity of water molecules (*arrow vectors*) due to impeding cellular density.

performed at low field strength, requires no post-processing, and is sensitive to local changes in molecular diffusivity.[5] Although not a common-place tool, it has some clinical utility in the setting of ultrafast MR imaging protocols for the detection of acute ischemic stroke.[6,7] Unfortunately, the interpretation of DWI with a single diffusion gradient must be limited to the direction that the gradient is applied[8] and is confounded by many other contrast mechanisms, including T1 and T2 relaxation.[9] These factors reduce its utility for head and neck imaging[4,5] (**Box 2**).

Apparent Diffusion Coefficient and Trace

Performing trace imaging with ADC mapping overcomes many shortcomings of conventional DWI (**Box 3**). Acquisition time remains relatively short, postprocessing is automated, and it does not require high-field-strength magnets. Images are obtained in at least 3 diffusion-sensitized directions and mathematically combined into a single trace sequence, which averages out any

directional dependence within the voxels. Many current MR imaging protocols perform diffusion imaging in at least 20 directions, creating a diffusion tensor (discussed later) that can be decomposed into isotropic and anisotropic components. The isotropic component represents the mean diffusivity (MD) when orientation is averaged. Thus, the diffusion trace image improves accuracy and signal-to-noise ratio by removing superimposed anisotropic structures (eg, white matter tracts).[4,5]

DWI trace is an intrinsically T2-weighted sequence. Therefore, signal intensity is influenced both by diffusion and T2 prolongation, which creates ambiguity when interpreting findings. To resolve this ambiguity, a map is created by combining information from the diffusion sequence with information from the same sequence performed without the diffusion gradients turned on. This mathematically removes the T2 effects, yielding a pure parametric diffusion image. Because this apparent diffusion coefficient (ADC) map is a calculated derivation of the different b value and directional images, however, artifacts and errors present in the measured data lead to decreased spatial resolution and signal-to-noise ratio compared with the trace image.[10]

ADC map combined with the trace sequence is highly sensitive in the detection of reduced diffusivity and central in the evaluation of ischemic stroke.[11] Increasingly, ADC and trace diffusion imaging are used in head and neck imaging, particularly in the assessment of benignity versus malignancy. As a generalization, malignant neoplasms demonstrate lower mean ADC values than benign tumors, owing to high cellularity, high nuclear-to-cytoplasmic ratio, and densely packed intracellular space. This is not infallible and exceptions to this rule commonly are encountered. Some benign lesions can demonstrate reduced diffusivity, yielding low mean ADC signal (eg, abscess, Warthin tumor, schwannoma, paraganglioma, meningioma, solitary fibrous tumor, cholesteatoma, hemangiopericytoma, and myoepithelial tumor)[12] (**Fig. 2**). Conversely, some low-cellularity malignant tumors, such as chondrosarcoma and chordoma, can have relatively high mean ADC values, mimicking benign lesions (**Fig. 3**). Despite its imperfections, many prior studies have shown DWI to be a promising tool for predicting malignant risk of head and lesions, the specificity of which may increase when performed in conjunction with other functional imaging techniques (eg, MR perfusion).[13–20]

Mean ADC values also have been used to predict histopathologic subtypes of some

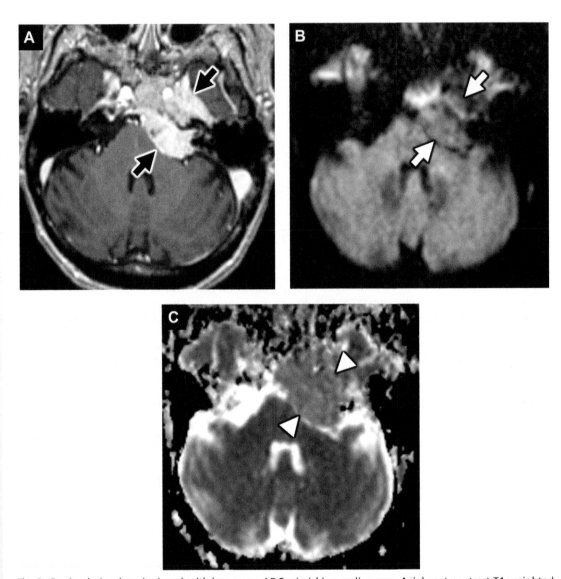

Fig. 2. Benign lesion (meningioma) with low mean ADC mimicking malignancy. Axial post-contrast T1-weighted imaging (A) shows an avidly enhancing mass (arrows) centered along the left petrous apex with extension into the sella, prepontine cistern, CPA, internal auditory canal, and middle cranial fossa with dural tail of enhancement typical of meningioma. Axial EPI DWI trace (B) shows the mass (arrows) to be mildly hyperintense with mean ADC approximating that of brain parenchyma. Axial ADC map (C) shows the mass to be hypointense (arrowheads) with mildly reduced diffusivity of water molecules due to relatively high cellularity of the meningioma.

malignancies. For example, human papilloma virus (HPV)-positive squamous cell carcinoma (SCC) has been shown to have lower mean ADC values than HPV-negative SCC.[21] Likewise, lymphoma often shows very low mean ADC values, which may help confer diagnostic confidence in distinguishing it from other intermediate and low-grade malignancies.[22,23] Mean ADC values also may be a sensitive and relatively specific tool for differentiating benign lymphadenopathy versus nodal metastasis in cancers, such as SCC and nasopharyngeal carcinoma, with metastatic nodes typically demonstrating lower ADC values than reactive nodes.[24–27] Even lower mean ADC values have been shown in nodal lymphoma,[28,29] which shows promise in conferring additional diagnostic value when evaluating for lymphoproliferative disorders. Emerging data suggest ADC/trace imaging may also prove a useful imaging biomarker for the prediction of HPV status in head and neck SCC nodal metastases, because HPV-positive metastatic lymph nodes demonstrate significantly

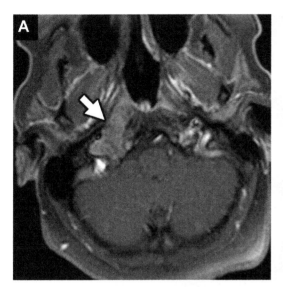
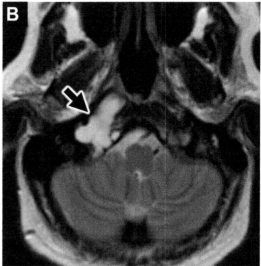

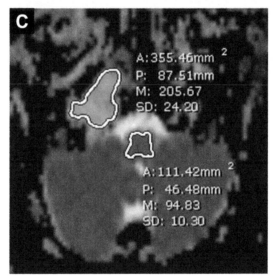

Fig. 3. Malignant lesion (chondrosarcoma) with high mean ADC mimicking benignity. Axial post-contrast T1-weighted imaging with fat saturation (A) shows a circumscribed right petrooccipital mass (arrow) with mild heterogeneous enhancement. Axial T2-weighted imaging (B) shows the mass (arrow) to be markedly hyperintense. Axial ADC map (C) shows the mass to be markedly hyperintense, with mean ADC more than 2-times greater than the medulla (lesion-to-medulla ADC$_{ratio}$ >2). Although increased ADC$_{ratio}$ is associated with higher likelihood of benignity,[41] chondrosarcoma is a prototypical outlier due to its low cellularity and frequent high mean ADC.

lower mean ADC values compared with HPV-negative metastatic nodes.[30]

DWI also has shown promise as a potential biomarker for assessing response to therapy in head and neck cancer. Prior studies have found that pretreatment tumors with necrosis and decreased vascularity have higher mean ADC values and generally are less responsive to chemotherapy and radiation therapy.[31,32] Furthermore, some studies have shown head and neck cancers with higher intratreatment and posttreatment ADC values demonstrate better overall survival and remission rates.[32–35] Other investigators have postulated that serial ADC measurements during the course of treatment may be useful in evaluating for treatment response, progression, and treatment resistance.[2]

In the postchemotherapy or radiation setting, patients manifest structural and molecular changes at the primary and nodal neoplastic sites that can make evaluation for recurrence challenging based on conventional MR sequences.

When treatment changes are confounding, DWI may confer additional predictive value and diagnostic specificity for tumor recurrence. In this regard, recurrent primary malignancy and metastatic nodal disease typically demonstrate lower mean ADC values than posttreatment changes and benign lymphoid tissue, respectively.[36,37]

Diffusion Tensor Imaging

DWI assumes water molecules move in all directions equally and uninhibited. Structural elements (eg, myelinated axons and cytoskeleton) in biologic tissue, however, inhibit or preferentially bias the direction of water movement. This directional preference, or anisotropy, can be imaged using a mathematical model called a tensor. Instead of a single value being assigned to a voxel, there are at least 6 values assigned to each voxel. The diffusion tensor usually is ellipsoid or cigar-shaped, giving the water molecules within a voxel a directional orientation. DTI allows measuring not only the magnitude (ADC value) but also the direction of diffusivity.[5] The most common metrics of DTI used are MD and fractional anisotropy (FA), which reflect the size (MD) and shape (FA) of the diffusion ellipsoids, respectively (Box 4).

DTI techniques may be used for tractography and neurography purposes, which may prove an emerging role in preoperative planning with respect to cranial nerves and brachial plexus. It also has been shown that FA value, like ADC, correlates with cellular density and may serve as a rough predictor for malignancy. Similarly, residual and recurrent cancers show lower MD values than post-treatment changes, due to high cellularity and lack of free water. The addition of FA and MD to mean ADC values has been shown to increase confidence in predicting primary and recurrent malignancy in the head and neck, but the role of these DTI parameters in clinical practice is not well established and probably should be regarded as an adjunct to routine pulse sequences and mean ADC[38,39] (Figs. 4 and 5).

Specific mean ADC thresholds for predicting benignity versus malignancy have been reported with DTI acquisition parameters, but imagers must recognize that such quantitative assessment is limited by variability across different MR systems and acquisition parameters.[40] It is critical to recognize that mean ADC values obtained with DTI parameters often are lower than mean ADC values obtained with DWI parameters—potentially below reported malignant DWI threshold values, which could result in false-positive examinations if DWI-specific thresholds are applied to DTI acquisitions.[41] As a workaround, it has been suggested that imagers use a normalized ADC ratio comparing the mean ADC of a lesion to that of an internal reference (eg, medulla or cervical spinal cord), thus normalizing ADC values across systems and across DWI versus DTI acquisitions[41] (see Fig. 5; Fig. 6).

Intravoxel Incoherent Motion

The gradient strength, duration of gradient, and interval between gradients determine how sensitive a sequence is to diffusion, and these diffusion effects can be interrogated at multiple b values. Fast-moving molecules lose signal because b values are increased at a much higher rate than slow-moving molecules; thus, as gradient strength increases, true brownian motion of water molecules dominates, leading to signal loss on diffusion images. At lower b values, a second diffusion mechanism contributes a small but measurable overall diffusion effect—microscopic perfusion due to microcirculation of water molecules in blood contained within the local capillary network. Because of the interplay between brownian motion effects at high b values and microperfusion effects at lower b values, free water loses nearly all signal at high b values (ie, b-1000 images demonstrate nulled cerebral spinal fluid) but maintains some signal intensity at lower b values (ie, b-0 images appear T2 weighted). These principles make up the core concept of intravoxel incoherent motion (IVIM), a technique that uses multiple different b values (0–1000 s/mm^2) to estimate tissue perfusion by exploiting differential signal loss seen at lower b values[42,43] (Box 5).

Box 4
Diffusion tensor imaging summary

Higher number of diffusion probing gradients than DWI

Mathematical model (tensor) of magnitude and direction of diffusivity

Resolves magnitude (ADC), size (MD), and shape (FA) of diffusion

Roles in tractography, neurography, and prediction of malignancy versus benignity

DTI-acquired mean ADC thresholds for predicting malignancy may differ from DWI-acquired thresholds

Many applications require postprocessing

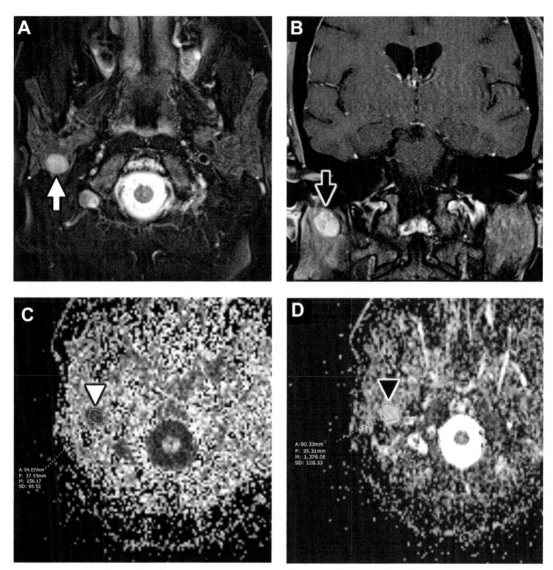

Fig. 4. Application of quantitative DTI parameters to predict benignity. Axial T2-weighted imaging with fat saturation (*A*) shows a circumscribed, relatively hyperintense right parotid mass (*arrow*), which is darker than cerebrospinal fluid. Coronal post-contrast T1-weighted imaging with fat saturation (*B*) shows the mass enhance avidly (*arrow*), but heterogeneously. The conventional sequences suggest benignity, but the T2 signal is darker than often is seen with pleomorphic adenoma, raising some concern for malignancy. Axial FA map (*C*) shows the mass to have markedly low FA (*arrowhead*), suggesting a low-cellularity tumor, a finding that is corroborated on axial ADC map (*D*) with marked hyperintense signal (*arrowhead*). Subsequent biopsy confirmed pleomorphic adenoma, a benign tumor.

Generally, IVIM has been used as an extension of DWI and ADC values as a marker for malignancy. By using a spectrum of b values, information pertaining to blood volume and blood flow can be obtained, thus acting as a surrogate for tissue perfusion and providing insight into tissue microvasculature. IVIM has proved useful for assessing tissue perfusion when contrast cannot be safely administered and has demonstrated fair to good correlation with other MR perfusion sequences.[42] Common metrics of IVIM include fractional diffusion (D_f or f), pure diffusion coefficient (D_{slow} or D), and pseudodiffusion coefficient (D_{fast} or D^*), although there are many parameters that may be assessed via this technique.[43]

IVIM has shown promise in head and neck oncologic imaging, but it is not yet a widely used application in routine clinical practice. Prior investigations of salivary gland tumors have

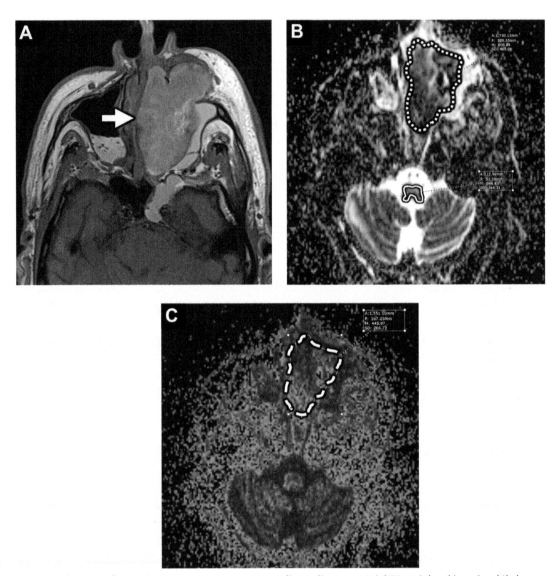

Fig. 5. Application of quantitative DTI parameters to predict malignancy. Axial T1-weighted imaging (*A*) shows a large, moderately hyperintense mass (*arrow*) involving the left maxillary sinus and nasal cavity, which obstructs the left maxillary and sphenoid sinuses and extends into the premaxillary soft tissues. Quantitative analysis of the ADC map (*B*) is performed as part of routine clinical workflow on PACS by drawing a freehand ROI around the lesion (*dotted line*) and medulla (*solid line*), sparing the peripheral 1 mm to 2 mm. In this case, the mean ADC value of the mass is 15% lower than that of the medulla (lesion-to-medulla ADC$_{ratio}$ = 0.85). A lesion-to-medulla ADC$_{ratio}$ less than 1 is associated with increased likelihood of malignancy.[41] This suspicion of malignancy also is corroborated on the axial FA map (*C*), which shows relatively high FA within the tumor (*dashed line*), suggesting increased cellularity. Subsequent biopsy demonstrated sinonasal melanoma.

shown that IVIM may help predict malignancy with malignant tumors demonstrating lower pure diffusion (D) than pleomorphic adenomas (albeit overlapping with Warthin tumors, a false-positive result if using the D parameter alone) and malignant tumors showing lower D* than Warthin tumors.[44,45] Other studies have evaluated the utility of IVIM in differentiating malignant from benign lesions outside the salivary glands with varying success. As a generalization, malignant lesions show lower D and D$_f$ values than benign lesions, with lymphoma typically significantly lower than other malignancies.[43,46] There is a growing body of evidence to suggest that IVIM-derived parameters may be a useful adjunct to ADC values when predicting tumor response to

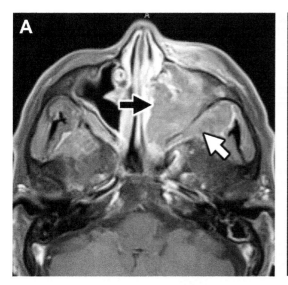

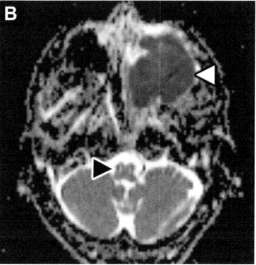

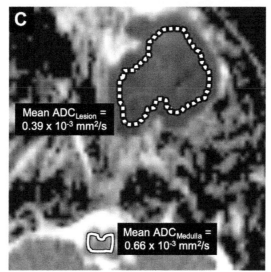

Fig. 6. Mean ADC value ROI evaluation for predicting malignancy. Axial post-contrast T1-weighted imaging with fat saturation (*A*) shows a hypoenhancing mass (*black arrow*) centered in the left maxillary sinus, which invades into the infrazygomatic masticator space (*white arrow*). Visual inspection of the ADC map (*B*) shows the mass (*white arrowhead*) to be markedly hypointense and lower in signal intensity than the medulla (*black arrowhead*). Quantitative analysis of the ADC map (*C*) is performed as per Fig. 5. In this case, the mean ADC value of the mass (*dotted line*) is approximately 40% lower (lesion-to-medulla ADC$_{ratio}$ = 0.59) than that of the medulla (*solid line*). A lesion-to-medulla ADC$_{ratio}$ less than 1 is associated with higher likelihood of malignancy.[41] Subsequent biopsy demonstrated sinonasal neuroendocrine carcinoma.

therapy, with D and D$_f$ demonstrating the greatest diagnostic accuracy.[47–49] There are conflicting data, however, regarding the utility of IVIM when evaluating response to therapy and tumor recurrence,[45] likely due in part to study heterogeneity and parameter selection.

Diffusion Kurtosis Imaging

Conventional DWI assumes that diffusion of free water follows a gaussian distribution with the signal monoexponentially decreasing as the b value increases. Due to the complex structure of most tissues, however, diffusion displacement varies from a gaussian form. The degree of deviation can be quantified using a dimensionless metric called diffusional kurtosis, which is regarded as a measure of a given tissue's degree of structure. In order to obtain the diffusional kurtosis, b values larger than those usually used in DWI (ie, >2000 s/mm²) are used so that the departure from linearity is apparent. Kurtosis (K) quantifies the deviation of tissue water molecules' diffusion from a gaussian distribution, whereas the diffusion coefficient (D) is the corrected diffusion coefficient for nongaussian bias.[50] Although still a nascent investigative technique that is not widely adopted for routine clinical practice, there have been studies demonstrating higher sensitivity of DKI than DWI for cancer detection, including studies demonstrating high sensitivity in the detection of malignant sinonasal lesions, nasopharyngeal carcinoma, parotid malignancy, and other malignant lesions of the head and neck[51–54] (Box 6).

PRACTICAL DIFFUSION-WEIGHTED IMAGING APPLICATIONS (LIFE HACKS) IN HEAD AND NECK IMAGING

Although some of the previously detailed diffusion variants (eg, DKI and IVIM) remain more in an investigative realm, the ubiquity of trace DWI and DTI parameters in neuroradiology practices warrants consideration of their roles in routine clinical head and neck imaging protocols. This section details several practical clinical applications that benefit from routine use of diffusion imaging as part of head and neck MR imaging protocols (Box 7).

Prediction of Benignity Versus Malignancy

Diffusion imaging can be a valuable adjunct to conventional MR imaging sequences for predicting the benignity versus malignancy of a head and neck mass. The authors acknowledge that this is an imperfect tool with recognized false-positive results, false-negative results, and technical differences in DWI sequences and MR imaging systems, yielding variability in quantitative DWI assessment between vendors and even between given vendors' scanner models. Nonetheless, the authors posit that DWI provides important, quantifiable data that, when taken into consideration with other clinicoradiologic features, often can increase confidence in the differentiation of benign versus malignant tumors in the head and neck. This quantitative assessment can be performed as part of routine clinical workflow by simple free-hand region-of-interest (ROI) analysis of target lesions within most picture archiving and communication system (PACS) software. Most investigators suggest constructing ROIs in the most solid or suspicious area of the mass or lymph node, sparing the peripheral 1 mm to 2 mm and avoiding cystic/necrotic portions when possible (see Fig. 6).

In general, malignant lesions tend to have lower mean ADC values compared with benign lesions. Using this framework, multiple prior investigations have put forth mean ADC thresholds for predicting benignity versus malignancy of head and neck lesions[15,29,41,55–59] (Table 1). The authors caution against relying absolutely on mean ADC thresholds, which are limited by heterogeneous sample populations in prior studies. Additionally, differences in scan parameters (eg, higher b values utilized in DTI vs DWI, matrix size, and magnetic field strength) and variability between scanners and manufacturers limit the reproducibility of

Table 1
Reported diffusion-weighted imaging and diffusion tensor imaging mean apparent diffusion coefficient values, thresholds, sensitivity, and specificity for benign and malignant lesions in the head and neck

Author	Field Strength (T)	Head and Neck Site	b Value (s/mm²)	Diffusion-Weighted Imaging vs Diffusion Tensor Imaging	Mean Apparent Diffusion Coefficient Value ± SD of Benign × 10⁻³ mm²/s	Mean Apparent Diffusion Coefficient Value ± SD of Malignant × 10⁻³ mm²/s	Malignant Threshold × 10⁻³ mm²/s	Sensitivity (%)	Specificity (%)
Wang et al,[59] 2001	1.5	Mixed	1000	DWI	1.56 ± 0.51	1.13 ± 0.43	<1.22	84	91
Bozgeyik et al,[15] 2009	1.5	Thyroid	300	DWI	1.15 ± 0.43	0.30 ± 0.20	<0.62	90	100
Sumi et al,[29] 2003	1.5	Metastatic lymph nodes	1000	DWI	0.30 ± 0.06	0.41 ± 0.10	>0.4	52	97
Sumi et al,[29] 2003	1.5	Lymphoma lymph nodes	1000	DWI	0.30 ± 0.06	022 ± 0.06	Unreported	Unreported	Unreported
de Bondt et al,[56] 2009	1.5	Metastatic lymph nodes	1000	DWI	1.2 ± 0.24	0.85 ± .19	<1.0	92	83
Srinivasan et al,[58] 2008	3	Mixed	1000	DWI	1.51 ± 0.487	1.07 ± 0.293	<1.3	Unreported	Unreported
Abdel Razek et al,[55] 2011	3	Orbit	1000	DWI	1.57 ± 0.33	0.84 ± 0.34	<1.15	95	91
Abdel Razek et al,[55] 2011	3	Skull base	1000	DWI	1.63 ± 0.29	1.00 ± 0.21	<1.3	94	93
Koontz & Wiggins,[41] 2017	Mixed (1.5 and 3)	Mixed	1000	DWI	1.43 ± 0.39	0.77 ± 0.53	<0.83	90	85
Koontz & Wiggins,[41] 2017	Mixed (1.5 and 3)	Mixed	2000	DTI	0.89 ± 29	0.55 ± 0.14	<0.7	91	74

Data from Refs.[15,29,41,55,56,58,59]

quantitative ADC measurement. To combat these variables, some investigators have suggested the use of an internal control (eg, medulla or spinal cord) to generate a normalized ADC ratio, which may be more reproducible between scanners and between DWI versus DTI parameters[41] (see **Figs. 5** and **6**).

Cholesteatoma

Cholesteatomas are non-neoplastic but locally destructive masslike accumulations of keratinizing squamous epithelium that may be congenital or acquired and occur most commonly in the middle ear.[60] Due to involvement of the conductive pathway, cholesteatomas are a common etiology for conductive hearing loss. High-resolution CT and MR imaging serve complementary roles in initial diagnosis, surgical planning, and postoperative follow-up of cholesteatoma.

Because of the nonspecific nature of temporal bone CT, MR imaging with DWI is a powerful tool

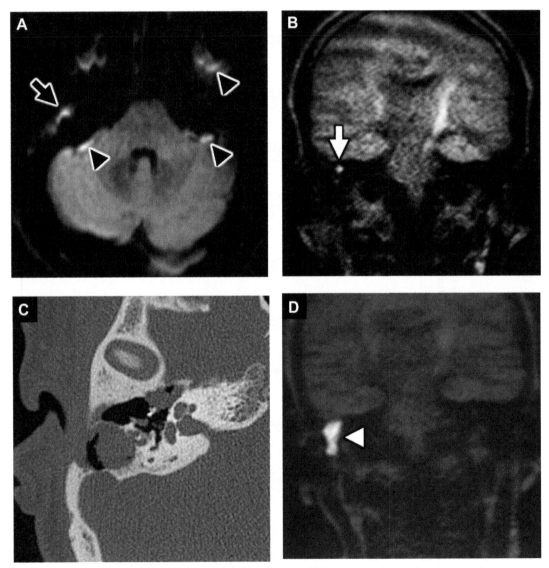

Fig. 7. DWI assessment of cholesteatoma. Axial EPI DWI trace (*A*) in a patient with questionable cholesteatoma shows bright signal in the right epitympanum (*arrow*), which is similar to susceptibility artifact (*arrowheads*) seen elsewhere and results in diagnostic ambiguity. Coronal non-EPI (HASTE) DWI (*B*) in the same patient confirms the presence of a small cholesteatoma (*arrow*) and is less affected by artifact. Axial non enhanced CT (*C*) of the temporal bones in a different patient shows lobular soft tissue in the mastoidectomy bowl, which may represent cholesteatoma or debris. Coronal non-EPI (HASTE) DWI (*D*) is helpful in definitively diagnosing recurrent cholesteatoma (*arrowhead*) in this postoperative setting.

for increasing diagnostic specificity. On MR imaging, cholesteatomas are characteristically isointense to hypointense on T1-weighted imaging, hyperintense on T2-weighted imaging, and nonenhancing with the exception of potential thin rind of surrounding enhancing granulation tissue.[60,61] DWI is invaluable in the assessment of cholesteatoma, because the keratin debris results in reduced diffusivity of water molecules, yielding markedly bright signal intensity on DWI trace[61,62] (Fig. 7).

Traditional echo planar imaging (EPI) DWI techniques have a lower sensitivity for detecting cholesteatoma than non-EPI DWI techniques, largely due to a combination of susceptibility, motion, and ghosting artifacts resulting from the single-shot spin-echo DWI pulse sequence used with EPI DWI.[62] Newer EPI DWI sequences using multishot or segmented EPI preparation (eg, RESOLVE [Siemens]) and small field-of-view DWI preparations (eg, ZOOMit [Siemens], FOCUS [GE], or iZOOM [Philips]) mitigate these artifacts and improve spatial resolution and signal-to-noise ratio constraints.[63] Non-EPI DWI sequences (eg, HASTE DWI) typically use a single-shot turbo-spin or multishot turbo-spin preparation with longer echo times, which reduce these artifacts and result in greater conspicuity of the cholesteatomas with the benefit of added spatial resolution and improved signal-to-noise ratio (see Fig. 7).

DWI also is valuable in screening postoperative patients for residual or recurrent cholesteatomas. In pooled meta-analysis, current non-EPI DWI was shown to have a sensitivity ranging between 86% and 93% and specificity ranging between 88% and 97% for detecting cholesteatoma.[64] Some investigators have concluded that current non-EPI DWI may obviate invasive second-look surgery, although this surveillance strategy remains controversial.[65]

Other Diffusion Trace-Bright Masses

Other masses or masslike lesions in the head and neck may be hyperintense on DWI trace sequences, including epidermoid cysts, meningiomas, chondrosarcomas, and chordomas. When a mass is found to be bright on the DWI trace, it is critical to further characterize the lesion on the ADC map to determine if the mass exhibits true reduced diffusivity (DWI trace bright + ADC dark, suggesting high cellularity) or is intrinsically T2 bright (DWI trace bright + ADC bright, suggesting low cellularity).

Epidermoid cysts histologically are akin to middle ear cholesteatomas but are found elsewhere in the body.[63] They are a relatively common cerebellopontine angle (CPA) mass but can be found in the cavernous sinus, orbits, and floor of mouth. On T2-weighted imaging, epidermoid cysts are markedly hyperintense and could be confused

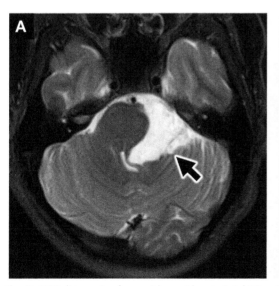
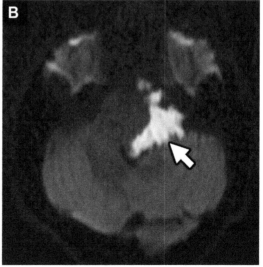

Fig. 8. DWI diagnosis of an epidermoid cyst. Axial T2-weighted imaging with fat saturation (A) shows an intrinsically T2 bright mass (arrow) centered in the left CPA, which exerts mass effect on the adjacent pons, superior and middle cerebellar peduncles, and cerebellum. Note a lack of edema within the pons and cerebellum, indicating a long-standing, slow-growing mass. Axial EPI DWI trace (B) shows marked signal hyperintensity (arrow) confirming the diagnosis of CPA epidermoid cyst.

for a CPA arachnoid cyst.[66] DWI is critical for making this diagnosis, because epidermoid cysts are markedly hyperintense on DWI trace with true reduced diffusivity[63,66,67] (Fig. 8).

Meningiomas typically are benign extra-axial neoplasms that may be relatively hyperintense on DWI trace due to increased cellularity (true reduced diffusivity) and/or a component of intrinsic increased T2 signal (T2 shine-through). Reduced diffusivity has been evaluated as a potential biomarker for atypical (World Health Organization grade II) or anaplastic (World Health Organization grade III) meningiomas,[68] which shows promise as a potential radiomics target

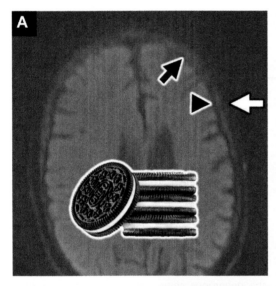

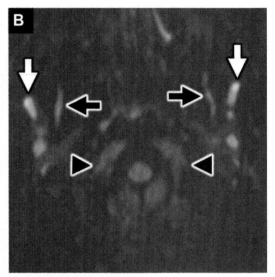

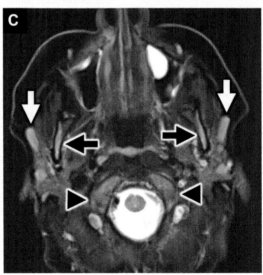

Fig. 9. DWI detection of marrow replacement. Axial EPI DWI trace (*A*) in an elderly patient imaged for stroke demonstrates markedly bright signal intensity within the marrow space of the calvarium (*black arrow*). This stands out against the nulled cerebrospinal fluid (*arrowhead*) and nulled subcutaneous fat signal (*white arrow*), giving the appearance of a Nabisco Oreo sandwich cookie (*inset*) viewed from side. In older patients, yellow (fatty) marrow that should be dark on EPI DWI from fat saturation is expected to be seen, but in this case has been replaced. Axial EPI DWI trace (*B*) and axial T2-weighted imaging with fat saturation (*C*) also show increased marrow signal intensity within the mandibles (*black arrows*) and occipital condyles (*arrowheads*) as well as hyperintense, enlarged intraparotid lymph nodes (*white arrows*) that stand out among the largely nulled extracranial soft tissues on EPI DWI trace. Subsequent marrow biopsy revealed chronic lymphocytic leukemia/small lymphocytic lymphoma.

in multiparametric meningioma grading.[69] Meningiomas of all grades may have reduced diffusivity and often stand out on DWI trace against the background brain parenchymal signal intensity and nulled marrow plus extracranial fat signal, making DWI trace a useful pulse sequence for meningioma detection—particularly if contrast cannot be given. Meningiomas also are a potential false-positive benign tumor with reduced diffusivity, which may be confused for a malignant lesion if the diffusion images are interpreted without consideration of the routine pulse sequences (see **Fig. 2**).

Two other head and neck tumors with frequent DWI trace hyperintensity are chondrosarcomas and chordomas, which are both relatively slow growing but malignant tumors encountered in the skull base. Unfortunately, chondrosarcomas and chordomas may have a similar appearance on conventional pulse sequences with characteristic bright T2 signal intensity and mild, often heterogeneous contrast enhancement. DWI may be

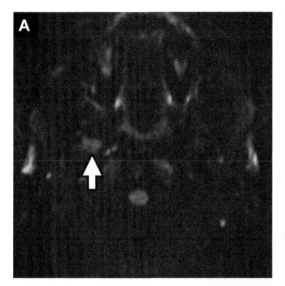
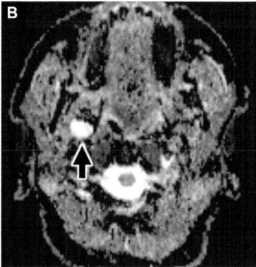
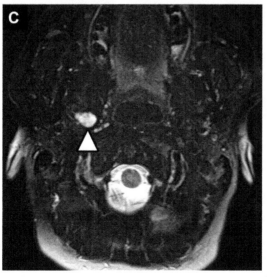

Fig. 10. DWI detection of incidental extracranial mass. Axial REadout Segmentation Of Long Variable Echo trains (RESOLVE) DWI trace (*A*) in a patient imaged for stroke symptoms shows a mildly hyperintense mass (*arrow*) in the deep lobe of the right parotid gland. Axial ADC map (*B*) shows even greater conspicuity of the hyperintense, low-cellularity mass (*arrow*). On axial T2-weighted imaging with fat saturation (*C*) the mass (*arrowhead*) is evident but less conspicuous than on ADC map (*B*). Subsequent biopsy confirmed pleomorphic adenoma.

a helpful adjunct sequence for differentiation, because chordomas are reported to have lower mean ADC values than chondrosarcomas.[70,71] Importantly, both chondrosarcoma and chordoma are relatively low-cellularity malignancies, often (if not usually) resulting in relatively bright ADC signal intensity that is greater than surrounding structures, including internal controls, such as the medulla (see **Fig. 3**). For this reason, chondrosarcomas and chordomas also are the prototypical false-negative malignant tumors with increased diffusivity (bright ADC signal) relative to brain parenchyma, which may be confused for benign lesions if too much emphasis is placed on the DWI sequences.

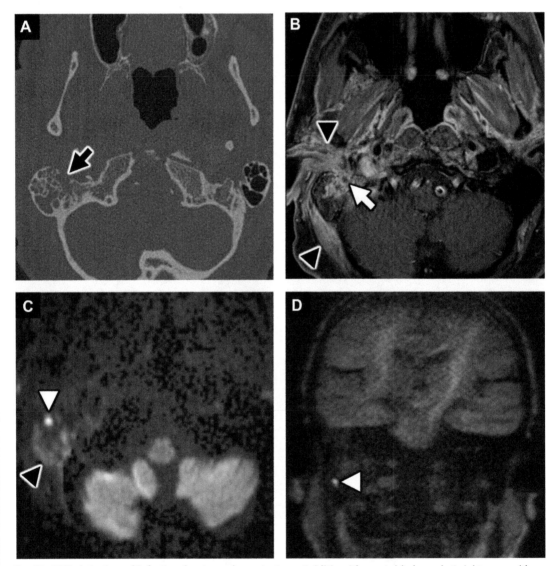

Fig. 11. DWI detection of infection (acute coalescent otomastoiditis with mastoid abscess). Axial temporal bone non enhanced CT (*A*) shows opacified right mastoid air cells with dehiscence of the cortex (*arrow*). Axial postcontrast T1-weighted imaging with fat saturation (*B*) demonstrates diffuse enhancement of the opacified mastoid air cells with enhancing phlegmon (*arrowheads*) in the surrounding soft tissues. Note a tiny focus of nonenhancement (*arrow*) at the focus of cortical dehiscence. Axial EPI DWI trace (*C*) shows lightbulb bright signal (*white arrowhead*) corresponding to the nonenhancing focus, indicating a small abscess. Note differential hyperintensity of the phlegmon (*black arrowhead*), which is less bright than the abscess. Coronal non-EPI (HASTE) DWI (*D*), which is less prone to artifact, confirms the tiny mastoid abscess (*arrowhead*) with reduced diffusivity. This case highlights the complementary role of CT and MR imaging in the assessment of acute otomastoiditis and associated complications.

Marrow Replacement

DWI can be a useful sequence for identifying marrow replacing processes, including neoplastic and infectious marrow etiologies. This is increasingly important given the growing use of volumetric T1-weighted sequences (eg, MPRAGE and SPGR), which are of limited assessment of marrow signal compared with traditional T1-weighted spin-echo sequences. Because EPI DWI sequences utilize a fat saturation preparation,

yellow marrow typical of middle-aged and older adults normally should be hypointense on DWI trace sequence. When the marrow space is infiltrated with a high-cellularity process (eg, leukemic marrow, cellular metastases, anemic red marrow reconversion, or marrow stem cell stimulation from granulocyte colony-stimulating factor administration) or edema (eg, osteomyelitis or metastases), an increase in marrow signal intensity (diffusion Oreo cookie sign) may be encountered on DWI trace (**Fig. 9**) that stands out against the

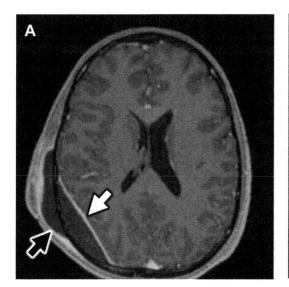
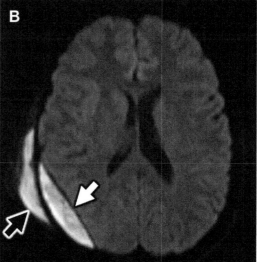
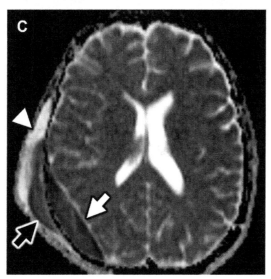

Fig. 12. DWI differentiation of abscess and phlegmon. Axial post-contrast T1 SPGR (*A*) in a child with acute coalescent otomastoiditis reveals large rim-enhancing fluid collections in the epidural (*white arrow*) and subgaleal (*black arrow*) spaces. These collections are markedly hyperintense on axial RESOLVE DWI trace (*B*) and hypointense on axial ADC map (*C*), confirming epidural (*white arrow*) and subgaleal (*black arrow*) abscesses. Note the signal hyperintensity throughout the overlying extracranial soft tissues (*arrowhead*) on ADC map (*C*), which helps differentiate the overlying phlegmon and edema from true abscess.

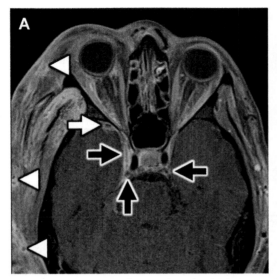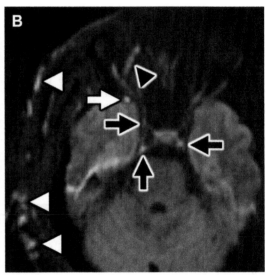

Fig. 13. DWI detection of septic thrombophlebitis. Axial post-contrast T1-weighted imaging with fat saturation (A) in an intravenous drug user shows diffuse edema and enhancement throughout the orbits, preorbital soft tissues, right face, and right masticator space consistent with cellulitis, phlegmon, and myositis. Subtle filling defects are seen within the expanded cavernous sinuses (*black arrows*), cortical veins (*white arrow*), and multiple superficial scalp veins (*arrowheads*), with surrounding enhancement due to septic thrombophlebitis. Against the dark background of the axial DTI trace (B), the numerous hyperintense thrombi within the cavernous sinuses (*black arrows*), cortical veins (*white arrow*), scalp veins (*white arrowheads*), and right superior ophthalmic vein (*black arrowhead*) are seen with much greater conspicuity.

dark background of intracranial cerebrospinal fluid and extracranial hypointense muscle and fat.[72,73]

Incidental Masses on Brain and Spine Imaging

DWI trace and ADC map acquired as part of routine brain and spine imaging often serve as useful tools to screen the included soft tissues of the neck for incidental masses. The differential T2 or diffusion signal intensity intrinsic to many masses relative to the background of dark (nulled fat) signal intensity seen within the soft tissues of the neck results in increased signal-to-noise ratio of lesions compared with the surrounding soft tissues (Fig. 10). Additionally, there are fewer visualized distractors (eg, vessels, muscle groups, and fat) on DWI trace and ADC than on conventional MR imaging sequences.

Infectious Processes

DWI can be a highly sensitive and in some cases specific technique for identifying certain infectious processes. For example, abscesses classically demonstrate internal reduced diffusivity (DWI trace bright and ADC dark) due to loculation of necrotic material rich in inflammatory cells, protein, debris, and bacteria that serve to limit the free diffusion of water molecules[74,75] (Figs. 11

and 12). Associated cellulitis and phlegmon also may be relatively bright on the DWI trace images but lack the marked ADC hypointensity characteristic of abscess, making diffusion imaging a particularly valuable tool in the diagnostic characterization of infection in the head and neck (see Fig. 12). Additionally, septic thrombophlebitis can be identified on DWI due to hyperintense signal of the necrotic material or intraluminal thrombus, depending on the ages of blood products within the clot (Fig. 13). Similarly, noninfectious vascular injury (eg, dissection or thrombosis) may be highly conspicuous on DWI trace (Fig. 14).

SUMMARY

Diffusion imaging provides many important insights into pathologies encountered in the head and neck. Although many of its roles remain investigative, a growing body of evidence supports its use as a valuable adjunct to conventional MR pulse sequences in the head and neck. Utilizing widely available clinical DWI and DTI sequences, radiologists can apply this complementary functional MR technique to many practical clinical applications, thus improving diagnostic sensitivity and specificity.

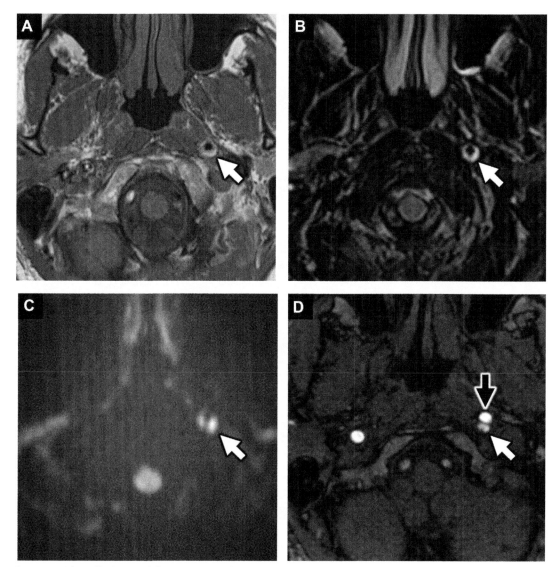

Fig. 14. Incidentally detected dissecting pseudoaneurysm on DWI. Axial T1-weighted MR imaging (*A*) in a patient imaged for hearing loss shows a subtle rim of bright signal intensity (*arrow*) eccentric to the left cervical internal carotid artery. Axial FLAIR MR imaging with fat saturation (*B*) shows increased signal within the mural hematoma (*arrow*), which mildly narrows the lumen. Axial EPI DWI trace (*C*) shows the mural thrombus to be markedly hyperintense (*arrow*) with tremendous conspicuity against the dark background from intrinsic fat saturation inherent in the EPI diffusion preparation. Follow-up axial time-of-flight MR angiogram (*D*) demonstrates an intimal flap with flow-related enhancement in the false lumen (*white arrow*) but maintained flow within the slightly narrowed true lumen (*black arrow*).

DISCLOSURE

The authors have nothing to disclose.

REFERENCES

1. El Beltagi AH, Elsotouhy AH, Own AM, et al. Functional magnetic resonance imaging of head and neck cancer: Performance and potential. Neuroradiol J 2019;32(1):36–52.

2. Thoeny HC. Diffusion-weighted MRI in head and neck radiology: applications in oncology. Cancer Imaging 2011;10:209–14.

3. Einstein A, Fürth R. Investigations on the theory of Brownian movement. New York: Dover Publications; 1956.

4. Bammer R. Basic principles of diffusion-weighted imaging. Eur J Radiol 2003;45(3):169–84.

5. Hagmann P, Jonasson L, Maeder P, et al. Understanding diffusion MR imaging techniques: from

scalar diffusion-weighted imaging to diffusion tensor imaging and beyond. Radiographics 2006;26(Suppl 1):S205–23.

6. U-King-Im JM, Trivedi RA, Graves MJ, et al. Utility of an ultrafast magnetic resonance imaging protocol in recent and semi-recent strokes. J Neurol Neurosurg Psychiatry 2005;76(7):1002–5.

7. Nael K, Khan R, Choudhary G, et al. Six-minute magnetic resonance imaging protocol for evaluation of acute ischemic stroke: pushing the boundaries. Stroke 2014;45(7):1985–91.

8. Le Bihan D, Urayama S, Aso T, et al. Direct and fast detection of neuronal activation in the human brain with diffusion MRI. Proc Natl Acad Sci U S A 2006; 103(21):8263–8.

9. Le Bihan D. Apparent diffusion coefficient and beyond: what diffusion MR imaging can tell us about tissue structure. Radiology 2013;268(2):318–22.

10. Minati L, Grisoli M, Bruzzone MG. MR spectroscopy, functional MRI, and diffusion-tensor imaging in the aging brain: a conceptual review. J Geriatr Psychiatry Neurol 2007;20(1):3–21.

11. Srinivasan A, Goyal M, Al Azri F, et al. State-of-the-art imaging of acute stroke. Radiographics 2006; 26(Suppl 1):S75–95.

12. Das A, Bhalla AS, Sharma R, et al. Benign neck masses showing restricted diffusion: Is there a histological basis for discordant behavior? World J Radiol 2016;8(2):174–82.

13. Yuan Y, Tang W, Jiang M, et al. Palatal lesions: discriminative value of conventional MRI and diffusion weighted imaging. Br J Radiol 2016;89(1059): 20150911.

14. Zheng N, Li R, Liu W, et al. The diagnostic value of combining conventional, diffusion-weighted imaging and dynamic contrast-enhanced MRI for salivary gland tumors. Br J Radiol 2018;91(1089): 20170707.

15. Bozgeyik Z, Coskun S, Dagli AF, et al. Diffusion-weighted MR imaging of thyroid nodules. Neuroradiology 2009;51(3):193–8.

16. El-Gerby KM, El-Anwar MW. Differentiating benign from malignant sinonasal lesions: feasibility of diffusion weighted MRI. Int Arch Otorhinolaryngol 2017; 21(4):358–65.

17. ElKhamary SM, Galindo-Ferreiro A, AlGhafri L, et al. Characterization of diffuse orbital mass using Apparent diffusion coefficient in 3-tesla MRI. Eur J Radiol Open 2018;5:52–7.

18. Tao X, Yang G, Wang P, et al. The value of combining conventional, diffusion-weighted and dynamic contrast-enhanced MR imaging for the diagnosis of parotid gland tumours. Dentomaxillofac Radiol 2017;46(6):20160434.

19. Yuan Y, Tang W, Tao X. Parotid gland lesions: separate and combined diagnostic value of conventional MRI, diffusion-weighted imaging and dynamic contrast-enhanced MRI. Br J Radiol 2016; 89(1060):20150912.

20. Sepahdari AR, Politi LS, Aakalu VK, et al. Diffusion-weighted imaging of orbital masses: multi-institutional data support a 2-ADC threshold model to categorize lesions as benign, malignant, or indeterminate. AJNR Am J Neuroradiol 2014;35(1): 170–5.

21. Driessen JP, van Bemmel AJ, van Kempen PM, et al. Correlation of human papillomavirus status with apparent diffusion coefficient of diffusion-weighted MRI in head and neck squamous cell carcinomas. Head Neck 2016;38(Suppl 1):E613–8.

22. Kato H, Kanematsu M, Watanabe H, et al. Differentiation of extranodal non-Hodgkins lymphoma from squamous cell carcinoma of the maxillary sinus: a multimodality imaging approach. Springerplus 2015;4:228.

23. Maeda M, Kato H, Sakuma H, et al. Usefulness of the apparent diffusion coefficient in line scan diffusion-weighted imaging for distinguishing between squamous cell carcinomas and malignant lymphomas of the head and neck. AJNR Am J Neuroradiol 2005;26(5):1186–92.

24. Jin GQ, Yang J, Liu LD, et al. The diagnostic value of 1.5-T diffusion-weighted MR imaging in detecting 5 to 10 mm metastatic cervical lymph nodes of nasopharyngeal carcinoma. Medicine (Baltimore) 2016; 95(32):e4286.

25. Vandecaveye V, De Keyzer F, Vander Poorten V, et al. Head and neck squamous cell carcinoma: value of diffusion-weighted MR imaging for nodal staging. Radiology 2009;251(1):134–46.

26. Payabvash S, Brackett A, Forghani R, et al. Differentiation of lymphomatous, metastatic, and non-malignant lymphadenopathy in the neck with quantitative diffusion-weighted imaging: systematic review and meta-analysis. Neuroradiology 2019; 61(8):897–910.

27. Chen C, Lin Z, Xiao Y, et al. Role of diffusion-weighted imaging in the discrimination of benign and metastatic parotid area lymph nodes in patients with nasopharyngeal carcinoma. Sci Rep 2018;8(1): 281.

28. Holzapfel K, Duetsch S, Fauser C, et al. Value of diffusion-weighted MR imaging in the differentiation between benign and malignant cervical lymph nodes. Eur J Radiol 2009;72(3):381–7.

29. Sumi M, Sakihama N, Sumi T, et al. Discrimination of metastatic cervical lymph nodes with diffusion-weighted MR imaging in patients with head and neck cancer. AJNR Am J Neuroradiol 2003;24(8): 1627–34.

30. Payabvash S, Chan A, Jabehdar Maralani P, et al. Quantitative diffusion magnetic resonance imaging for prediction of human papillomavirus status in head and neck squamous-cell carcinoma: A

systematic review and meta-analysis. Neuroradiol J 2019;32(4):232–40.

31. Razek AA, Megahed AS, Denewer A, et al. Role of diffusion-weighted magnetic resonance imaging in differentiation between the viable and necrotic parts of head and neck tumors. Acta Radiol 2008;49(3): 364–70.

32. King AD, Chow KK, Yu KH, et al. Head and neck squamous cell carcinoma: diagnostic performance of diffusion-weighted MR imaging for the prediction of treatment response. Radiology 2013;266(2):531–8.

33. Kim S, Loevner L, Quon H, et al. Diffusion-weighted magnetic resonance imaging for predicting and detecting early response to chemoradiation therapy of squamous cell carcinomas of the head and neck. Clin Cancer Res 2009;15(3):986–94.

34. King AD, Mo FK, Yu KH, et al. Squamous cell carcinoma of the head and neck: diffusion-weighted MR imaging for prediction and monitoring of treatment response. Eur Radiol 2010;20(9):2213–20.

35. Vandecaveye V, Dirix P, De Keyzer F, et al. Predictive value of diffusion-weighted magnetic resonance imaging during chemoradiotherapy for head and neck squamous cell carcinoma. Eur Radiol 2010;20(7): 1703–14.

36. Abdel Razek AA, Kandeel AY, Soliman N, et al. Role of diffusion-weighted echo-planar MR imaging in differentiation of residual or recurrent head and neck tumors and posttreatment changes. AJNR Am J Neuroradiol 2007;28(6):1146–52.

37. Vandecaveye V, De Keyzer F, Nuyts S, et al. Detection of head and neck squamous cell carcinoma with diffusion weighted MRI after (chemo)radiotherapy: correlation between radiologic and histopathologic findings. Int J Radiat Oncol Biol Phys 2007;67(4): 960–71.

38. Abdel Razek AAK. Diffusion tensor imaging in differentiation of residual head and neck squamous cell carcinoma from post-radiation changes. Magn Reson Imaging 2018;54:84–9.

39. Yu J, Du Y, Lu Y, et al. Application of DTI and ARFI imaging in differential diagnosis of parotid tumours. Dentomaxillofac Radiol 2016;45(6):20160100.

40. Connolly M, Srinivasan A. Diffusion-weighted imaging in head and neck cancer: technique, limitations, and applications. Magn Reson Imaging Clin N Am 2018;26(1):121–33.

41. Koontz NA, Wiggins RH 3rd. Differentiation of benign and malignant head and neck lesions with diffusion tensor imaging and DWI. AJR Am J Roentgenol 2017;208(5):1110–5.

42. Federau C. Intravoxel incoherent motion MRI as a means to measure in vivo perfusion: A review of the evidence. NMR Biomed 2017;30(11). https://doi.org/10.1002/nbm.3780.

43. Noij DP, Martens RM, Marcus JT, et al. Intravoxel incoherent motion magnetic resonance imaging in head and neck cancer: A systematic review of the diagnostic and prognostic value. Oral Oncol 2017; 68:81–91.

44. Sumi M, Van Cauteren M, Sumi T, et al. Salivary gland tumors: use of intravoxel incoherent motion MR imaging for assessment of diffusion and perfusion for the differentiation of benign from malignant tumors. Radiology 2012;263(3):770–7.

45. Sasaki M, Sumi M, Eida S, et al. Simple and reliable determination of intravoxel incoherent motion parameters for the differential diagnosis of head and neck tumors. PLoS One 2014;9(11):e112866.

46. Sumi M, Nakamura T. Head and neck tumors: assessment of perfusion-related parameters and diffusion coefficients based on the intravoxel incoherent motion model. AJNR Am J Neuroradiol 2013;34(2):410–6.

47. Guo W, Luo D, Lin M, et al. Pretreatment intra-voxel incoherent motion diffusion-weighted imaging (IVIM-DWI) in predicting induction chemotherapy response in locally advanced hypopharyngeal carcinoma. Medicine (Baltimore) 2016;95(10):e3039.

48. Hauser T, Essig M, Jensen A, et al. Prediction of treatment response in head and neck carcinomas using IVIM-DWI: Evaluation of lymph node metastasis. Eur J Radiol 2014;83(5):783–7.

49. Paudyal R, Oh JH, Riaz N, et al. Intravoxel incoherent motion diffusion-weighted MRI during chemoradiation therapy to characterize and monitor treatment response in human papillomavirus head and neck squamous cell carcinoma. J Magn Reson Imaging 2017;45(4):1013–23.

50. Jensen JH, Helpern JA, Ramani A, et al. Diffusional kurtosis imaging: the quantification of non-gaussian water diffusion by means of magnetic resonance imaging. Magn Reson Med 2005;53(6):1432–40.

51. Jiang JX, Tang ZH, Zhong YF, et al. Diffusion kurtosis imaging for differentiating between the benign and malignant sinonasal lesions. J Magn Reson Imaging 2017;45(5):1446–54.

52. Yuan J, Yeung DK, Mok GS, et al. Non-Gaussian analysis of diffusion weighted imaging in head and neck at 3T: a pilot study in patients with nasopharyngeal carcinoma. PLoS One 2014;9(1):e87024.

53. Minosse S, Marzi S, Piludu F, et al. Correlation study between DKI and conventional DWI in brain and head and neck tumors. Magn Reson Imaging 2017;42:114–22.

54. Qian W, Xu XQ, Zhu LN, et al. Preliminary study of using diffusion kurtosis imaging for characterizing parotid gland tumors. Acta Radiol 2019;60(7):887–94.

55. Abdel Razek A, Mossad A, Ghonim M. Role of diffusion-weighted MR imaging in assessing malignant versus benign skull-base lesions. Radiol Med 2011;116(1):125–32.

56. de Bondt RB, Hoeberigs MC, Nelemans PJ, et al. Diagnostic accuracy and additional value of

diffusion-weighted imaging for discrimination of malignant cervical lymph nodes in head and neck squamous cell carcinoma. Neuroradiology 2009; 51(3):183–92.

57. Razek AA, Elkhamary S, Mousa A. Differentiation between benign and malignant orbital tumors at 3-T diffusion MR-imaging. Neuroradiology 2011;53(7): 517–22.

58. Srinivasan A, Dvorak R, Perni K, et al. Differentiation of benign and malignant pathology in the head and neck using 3T apparent diffusion coefficient values: early experience. AJNR Am J Neuroradiol 2008; 29(1):40–4.

59. Wang J, Takashima S, Takayama F, et al. Head and neck lesions: characterization with diffusion-weighted echo-planar MR imaging. Radiology 2001;220(3):621–30.

60. Schwartz KM, Lane JI, Bolster BD Jr, et al. The utility of diffusion-weighted imaging for cholesteatoma evaluation. AJNR Am J Neuroradiol 2011;32(3): 430–6.

61. Dremmen MH, Hofman PA, Hof JR, et al. The diagnostic accuracy of non-echo-planar diffusion-weighted imaging in the detection of residual and/or recurrent cholesteatoma of the temporal bone. AJNR Am J Neuroradiol 2012;33(3):439–44.

62. Fischer N, Schartinger VH, Dejaco D, et al. Readout-segmented echo-planar DWI for the detection of cholesteatomas: correlation with surgical validation. AJNR Am J Neuroradiol 2019;40(6):1055–9.

63. Jambawalikar S, Liu MZ, Moonis G. Advanced MR imaging of the temporal bone. Neuroimaging Clin N Am 2019;29(1):197–202.

64. Lingam RK, Bassett P. A meta-analysis on the diagnostic performance of non-echoplanar diffusion-weighted imaging in detecting middle ear cholesteatoma: 10 years on. Otol Neurotol 2017;38(4): 521–8.

65. Horn RJ, Gratama JWC, van der Zaag-Loonen HJ, et al. Negative predictive value of non-echo-planar diffusion weighted MR imaging for the detection of residual cholesteatoma done at 9 months after primary surgery is not high enough to omit second look surgery. Otol Neurotol 2019;40(7):911–9.

66. Sirin S, Gonul E, Kahraman S, et al. Imaging of posterior fossa epidermoid tumors. Clin Neurol Neurosurg 2005;107(6):461–7.

67. Bergui M, Zhong J, Bradac GB, et al. Diffusion-weighted images of intracranial cyst-like lesions. Neuroradiology 2001;43(10):824–9.

68. Liu Y, Chotai S, Chen M, et al. Preoperative radiologic classification of convexity meningioma to predict the survival and aggressive meningioma behavior. PLoS One 2015;10(3):e0118908.

69. Laukamp KR, Shakirin G, Baessler B, et al. Accuracy of radiomics-based feature analysis on multi-parametric magnetic resonance images for noninvasive meningioma grading. World Neurosurg 2019;132:e366–90.

70. Welzel T, Meyerhof E, Uhl M, et al. Diagnostic accuracy of DW MR imaging in the differentiation of chordomas and chondrosarcomas of the skull base: A 3.0-T MRI study of 105 cases. Eur J Radiol 2018; 105:119–24.

71. Yeom KW, Lober RM, Mobley BC, et al. Diffusion-weighted MRI: distinction of skull base chordoma from chondrosarcoma. AJNR Am J Neuroradiol 2013;34(5):1056–61. S1051.

72. Cao W, Liang C, Gen Y, et al. Role of diffusion-weighted imaging for detecting bone marrow infiltration in skull in children with acute lymphoblastic leukemia. Diagn Interv Radiol 2016;22(6):580–6.

73. Padhani AR, Koh DM, Collins DJ. Whole-body diffusion-weighted MR imaging in cancer: current status and research directions. Radiology 2011; 261(3):700–18.

74. Bhatt N, Gupta N, Soni N, et al. Role of diffusion-weighted imaging in head and neck lesions: Pictorial review. Neuroradiol J 2017;30(4):356–69.

75. Kito S, Morimoto Y, Tanaka T, et al. Utility of diffusion-weighted images using fast asymmetric spin-echo sequences for detection of abscess formation in the head and neck region. Oral Surg Oral Med Oral Pathol Oral Radiol Endod 2006;101(2):231–8.

Magnetic Resonance Spectroscopy of the Head and Neck
Principles, Applications, and Challenges

Noriyuki Fujima, MD, PhD[a,b,1], V. Carlota Andreu-Arasa, MD, PhD[a,1],
Glenn D. Barest, MD[a,1], Ashok Srinivasan, MD, DNB[c],
Osamu Sakai, MD, PhD[a,d,e],*

KEYWORDS

- [1]H-magnetic resonance spectroscopy • ^{31}P-magnetic resonance spectroscopy
- Head and neck tumor • Choline/creatine (Cho/Cr) ratio

KEY POINTS

- Cho/Cr ratio may be a useful tool to differentiate malignant neoplastic lesions from benign lesions and normal tissues.
- There is still no clear evidence for the utility of pretreatment ^{1}H-MRS evaluation to predict treatment outcome in patients with head and neck cancers.
- The presence of Cho peak in post-treatment tissues has high specificity for residual or recurrent head and neck cancers.
- Compared with ^{1}H-MRS, there have been very limited studies of ^{31}P-MRS studies in the head and neck.
- Although the technique has potential, the clinical utility of ^{31}P-MRS has not yet been proven.

INTRODUCTION

Functional information derived from MR imaging reflects the biological characteristics of tissue and is reported to be important for the assessment of head and neck lesions.[1–6] Magnetic resonance spectroscopy (MRS) is a noninvasive technique that can provide functional information through the evaluation of tissue metabolite concentrations. Tissue metabolite detection is achieved by measuring signal of MR spectrum with different frequencies within a specific voxel set in the target tissue. In this process, the acquired MRS signal data are postprocessed with Fourier transformation technique, and the MR spectrum of signal amplitude with the resonant frequencies described by parts per million (ppm) is obtained. Proton MRS (^{1}H-MRS) has been widely used to evaluate the brain and lesions of the central nervous system since the 1980s. More recently, interest has turned toward the development of this

[a] Department of Radiology, Boston Medical Center, Boston University School of Medicine, One Boston Medical Center Place, Boston, MA 02118, USA; [b] Research Center for Cooperative Projects, Hokkaido University Graduate School of Medicine, kita 15, nishi 7, kita-ku, Sapporo, Hokkaido 060-8638, Japan; [c] Department of Radiology, Michigan Medicine, 1500 East Medical Center Drive B2-A209A, Ann Arbor, MI 48109, USA; [d] Department of Radiation Oncology, Boston Medical Center, Boston University School of Medicine, One Boston Medical Center Place, Boston, MA 02118, USA; [e] Department of Otolaryngology–Head and Neck Surgery, Boston Medical Center, Boston University School of Medicine, One Boston Medical Center Place, Boston, MA 02118, USA
[1] Present address: 820 Harrison Avenue, Boston, MA.
* Corresponding author. Department of Radiology, Boston Medical Center, Boston University School of Medicine, 820 Harrison Avenue, FGH Building 3rd Floor, Boston, MA 02118.
E-mail address: osamu.sakai@bmc.org

Neuroimag Clin N Am 30 (2020) 283–293
https://doi.org/10.1016/j.nic.2020.04.006

application in the evaluation of head and neck lesions. As in brain imaging, ^{1}H-MRS is the most commonly used spectroscopy technique for the evaluation of head and neck lesions. The metabolites detected by ^{1}H-MRS in head and neck lesions mainly include choline (Cho), creatine (Cr), lipid (Lip), and lactate (Lac). Several investigations have also reported use of phosphorus MRS (^{31}P-MRS). Different metabolic activities are originated from different physiologic and pathologic characteristics. Tissue metabolic activities obtained from MRS can be clinically useful to evaluate the characteristics in head and neck lesions.

MAGNETIC RESONANCE IMAGING PROTOCOL
Target Tissue Selection

Spectroscopic evaluation of tissue metabolites can be performed using 2 methods—single-voxel and multivoxel chemical shift imaging (CSI) techniques. Most published MRS reports in the head and neck have used single-voxel technique, which targets a tissue volume of interest (VOI) with one voxel, often measuring between 1 and 8 cm^3. The VOI should be placed within the lesion to avoid contamination by signal from adjacent tissues. Because signal-to-noise ratio (SNR) is generally considered to be proportional to voxel size, use of larger voxel sizes results in higher SNR but however risks contamination by soft tissues outside the lesion. Three-plane (axial, coronal, and sagittal) T1- or T2-weighted images are often acquired as a reference for VOI placement. Adequate VOI placement in the head and neck is challenging because lesions are often small, heterogeneous, poorly defined, and surrounded by complex anatomy. VOI selection by a radiologist familiar with head and neck imaging is highly recommended. Representative VOI placement in the neck is shown in **Fig. 1**.

Image Acquisition: Point-Resolved Spectroscopy or Stimulated Echo Acquisition Mode

Two major sequence designs are used in MRS signal acquisition: point-resolved spectroscopy (PRESS) and stimulated echo acquisition mode (STEAM). PRESS uses a double spin-echo sequence with 3 slice-selective pulses in orthogonal planes (ie, 90° excitation pulse, followed by two 180° slice-selective radiofrequency pulses). STEAM uses 3 orthogonally slice-selective 90° pulses (ie, 3 times 90° radiofrequency pulses). PRESS can be acquired with high SNR (two times higher than STEAM); however, the specific absorption rate, a measure of the rate at which energy is absorbed by the body, is also higher because of the use of 2 180° pulses. In contrast, STEAM uses stimulated echo with slice-selective 90° pulses that result in lower SNR. The shorter echo time (TE) setting possible with the STEAM method allows for detection of metabolites with short T2 times (eg, several kinds of amino acids such as glutamine or glutamate). Basic characteristics of PRESS and STEAM are summarized in **Table 1**. Scan times depend on several parameters, including field strength, voxel size, and the number of excitations, usually able to provide adequate spectra in the range of 5 to 10 minutes per VOI.

Water and Fat Suppression

Suppression of the abundant signals from water and fat is generally required to detect tissue metabolites in the clinical ^{1}H-MRS procedure.

Water suppression
In ^{1}H-MRS, the concentration of protons related to target metabolites is very small compared with that of bulk water (on the order of 1×10^{-3}M); therefore, suppression of signal due to water is crucial to obtain appropriate spectra. Several methods have been developed to suppress the water resonance. The most commonly used technique is a frequency selective pulse (4.7 ppm) applied before the excitation pulse. Only water spins receive an excitation pulse into the transverse plane (others remain along the z-axis), then a crusher gradient pulse is applied to dephase water spins.[7]

Fat suppression
Large lipid peaks result from the abundant adipose tissue in the neck. The large lipid peak may distort the spectral baseline and limit the detection of certain metabolites. Lipids should be suppressed using outer volume suppression techniques. Usually, the signal saturation of bulk fat is performed using a chemical shift selective imaging sequence pulse, which cancels the lipid signal by using the intrinsic chemical shift difference between lipid and water protons.

Shimming

Acquisition of appropriate MRS signal data of the lesion is technically challenging in the head and neck. Various artifacts arising from the complex anatomy of the head and neck, as well as air in the vicinity of the target lesion, and patient motion from breathing or swallowing may significantly reduce the SNR in MRS data. Adequate shimming is important to reduce magnetic field inhomogeneity and to maintain the well-balance of the magnetic field by adjusting the electric currents in the

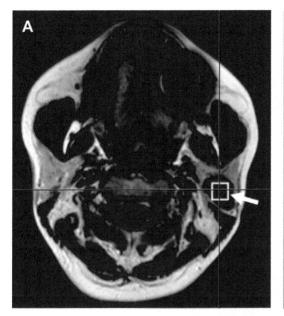
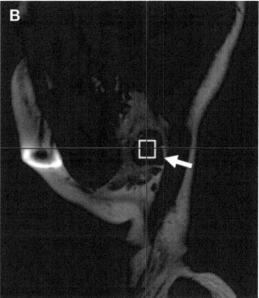

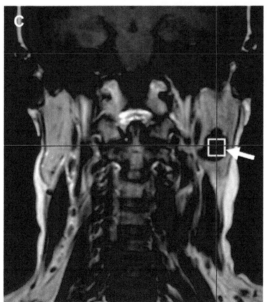

Fig. 1. Placement of target VOI. T1-weighted images in orthogonal planes—(A): axial, (B): coronal, and (C): sagittal—were used as reference images for VOI placement in a tumor of the left parotid gland. VOI placement should be carefully performed to include the target lesion and avoid surrounding normal tissue and MR signal contamination (A, B, and C, arrows). Red lines indicate the intersecting planes.

linear x-, y-, and z-gradient coils. If the scanner allows, high-order shimming that modifies more spatially complex magnetic field inhomogeneities should be performed. Manual volume shimming of the region encompassing the target VOI will also be required. Inappropriate shimming usually results in inaccurate signal acquisition (eg, shifts of peaks, contamination of peaks, and elevation of baseline noise).[8]

Postprocessing

Postprocessing of ^{1}H-MRS requires various types of algorithms to treat the raw data, such as zero-filling, line broadening, eddy current corrections, Fourier transformation, phasing, baseline correction, peak fitting, and intensity and area approximations. With current clinical scanners, many of these postprocessing tasks have been automated

Table 1
Comparison of point-resolved spectroscopy and stimulated echo acquisition mode

Techniques	PRESS	STEAM
TR	1500–2000 ms	1500–2000 ms
TE	135 or 270 ms	35 ms
Readout	90-180-180 (spin echo)	90-90-90 (stimulated echo)
Advantage	High SNR	Low SAR, setting of short TE
Disadvantage	High SAR	Low SNR

Abbreviation: SAR, specific absorption rate.

and produce accurate spectra and ratios of metabolites.

METABOLIC ACTIVITY

In head and neck lesions, the metabolites Cho, Cr, Lip, and Lac are often evaluated by ^{1}H-MRS.

1. *Choline*: the peak of Cho appears at 3.2 ppm. Cho is one of the phospholipid metabolites associated with cell membranes. It is considered to have a relationship with increased turnover of cell membranes, which reflects active cellular proliferation.
2. *Creatine*: the peak of Cr appears at 3.0 ppm. Cr reflects the energetic systems and intracellular metabolism. The concentration of Cr is maintained as a constant, and it is generally considered a stable metabolite. Therefore, the Cr peak is usually regarded as an internal reference for measuring changes in other metabolite peaks, especially Cho.
3. *Lipids*: usually, Lip components of cell membranes are not identified unless very short TE (30 or 35 ms) is used. Two peaks of lipids are generally observed at 1.3 ppm (methylene protons) and at 0.9 ppm (methyl protons). Lipid peaks can be observed in certain conditions, for example, primary or metastatic malignant tumors secondary to cellular membrane breakdown or necrosis.[9] Artifactual lipid peaks may be demonstrated if the voxel is inappropriately placed due to contamination from adjacent adipose tissues.
4. *Lactate*: the Lac peak is observed as a doublet at 1.33 ppm. This peak may result from anaerobic glycolysis, such as from hypoxic conditions in cancerous tissue. The peak of Lac is very close to that of Lip, thus separate quantitation of these 2 peaks may be impossible using some techniques. However, the Lac peak is inverted below the baseline within a certain range of TEs (TE = 135–144 ms). Therefore, with the optimal selection of TE parameter, the presence of Lac can be successfully discriminated.
5. *Other important metabolites*: several other amino acids, such as glutamine (Gln) and glutamate (Glu), or the combined Gln + Glu + gamma amino butyric acid described as Glx, with peaks in the range of 2.2 to 2.4 ppm have been reported in head and neck squamous cell carcinomas (HNSCC).[10]

Representative ^{1}H-MRS peaks of a recurrent HNSCC are presented in **Fig. 2**.

CLINICAL UTILITY
Differentiation of Benign and Malignant Lesions and Normal Tissue

Head and neck tumors; comparison to normal tissue
Several MRS studies, both in vivo and in vitro, have demonstrated differences between HNSCCs and normal muscles.[11–15] In those studies, the Cho/Cr ratio was significantly elevated in cancer tissues in comparison to normal neck musculature. Cho/Cr ratios with acquisition TE of 135 ms were 1.5–4.0 for HNSCCs, and 0–2.0 for normal neck muscles. Most studies concluded that the elevated Cho/Cr ratios for HNSCC were due to increased cell membrane turnover in the cancer tissue. Cho/Cr ratio was described to be increased with elevated TEs due to the short T2 relaxation time of Cr.[11,12] In addition to HNSCC, thyroid cancers have been distinguished from normal thyroid tissue based on the presence of Cho in the spectra.[16] In terms of comparison between malignant and inflammatory lesions in the neck, Yu and colleagues[17] reported markedly higher Cho peaks in malignant lesions than in chronic infections in various locations.

Head and neck tumors: comparison between benign and malignant lesions
Metabolite analysis in benign and malignant head and neck lesions has been described in several studies.[13,14,18] Surprisingly, previous reports described Cho/Cr ratio to be significantly higher in benign tumors compared with

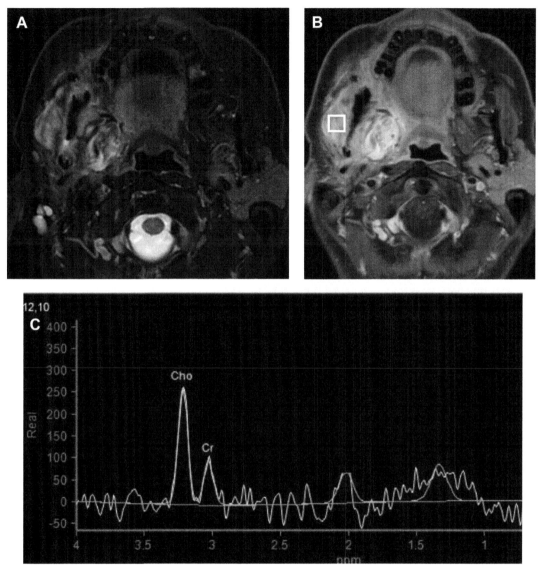

Fig. 2. ¹H-MRS in a recurrent SCC. Axial T2-weighted (A) and postcontrast T1-weighted (B) images in a 58-year-old man with a history of treated oral cavity SCC demonstrates new heterogeneous T2 hyperintensity and enhancement within the right masticator space. A VOI has been placed over the right masseter muscle. The corresponding ¹H-MRS spectrum (C) shows an elevated Choline peak in this pathologically proven recurrent SCC.

malignant tumors. Shailendra and colleagues reported the higher Cho/Cr ratio in benign tumors (inverted papillomas, glomus tumors, and schwannomas; Cho/Cr ratio of 2.2–5.55 with TE 136 ms) than in HNSCCs (Cho/Cr ratio of 0.82–3.84 with TE 136 ms). This relatively higher Cho/Cr ratio of benign tumors was thought to be due to neoplastic cellular proliferation,[13] analogous to the presence of elevated Cho/Cr ratio in intracranial meningiomas. Similarly, previous studies have demonstrated higher Cho/Cr ratios in meningiomas compared with high-grade gliomas.[1,19]

Subsequently, another study showed the same tendency with the following results: Cho/Cr ratio with TE 135 ms in benign tumors (24.4, range 1.4–59.7) was greater than malignant tumors (5.2, range 1.7–17.8).[20] Yu and colleagues also evaluated the Cho peaks among various maxillofacial and neck benign tumors in another report. They detected a Cho peak in some solid tumors (eg, pleomorphic adenoma, Warthin tumor, schwannoma, etc.) and noted absence of a Cho peak in most of cystic lesions (eg, lymphangioma, cyst, hemangioma, etc.).[18]

Salivary gland lesions

In parotid gland tumors, significantly higher Cho/Cr ratios have been reported in benign tumors (Warthin tumors, pleomorphic adenomas, and oncocytoma) compared with malignant tumors. In addition, significantly higher Cho/Cr ratios have been reported in Warthin tumors compared with pleomorphic adenomas.[21] In this report, the investigators discussed the cause of elevated Cho/Cr ratio in the tumor tissue was due to hypercellularity and inflammatory process; higher Cho/Cr ratio in Warthin tumors was thought to be due to a higher number of lymphocytes in the histopathology compared with other tumors. They reported the Cho/Cr ratio with TE 136 ms scanning was 5.49 ± 1.86 in Warthin tumors, 3.46 ± 0.84 in pleomorphic adenomas, 2.45 (only one case) in oncocytoma, and 1.73 ± 0.47 in malignant tumors. These results seem promising; however, they also reported measurable signal of Cho/Cr was recognized in only 47% of included parotid tumors. Yu and colleagues[18] investigated the detection rate of Cho peak in benign maxillofacial and neck lesions including parotid gland tumors; a higher detection rate of Cho peak was observed in Warthin tumors (5 of 7 cases, 71.4%) than pleomorphic adenomas (3 of 8 cases, 37.5%). In recent report by Zhu and colleagues,[22] Cho detection rate was useful for the differentiation of the mucosa-associated lymphoid tissue lymphoma (16 of 20 cases, 80%) and tumorlike benign lymphoepithelial lesion (6 of 19 cases, 24%).

Thyroid lesions

Several studies have investigated MRS findings in malignant and benign thyroid nodules.[23–25] In an early report by Gupta and colleagues,[23] the presence of a Cho peak in the targeted thyroid nodule had perfect sensitivity (100%) and high specificity (88.8%) for detection of malignancy. A recent report by Aghaghazvini and colleagues[25] has demonstrated a higher ratio of Cho/Cr in malignant thyroid tumors compared with benign nodules (6.6 ± 5.3 vs 0.8 ± 0.6, respectively, using TE 136 ms) at 3.0 T. The opposite tendency of Cho/Cr ratio in relation to benign versus malignant tumors is reported for parotid versus thyroid glands, which could be due to the difference of pathologies at the different primary sites.

Lymph node evaluation

Regarding lymph node evaluation, a pilot study from King and colleagues[26] analyzed the Cho/Cr ratio in a small cohort with various pathologies including both malignant (SCC, undifferentiated carcinoma, and lymphoma) and benign (tuberculosis and Castleman disease) nodal diseases

(Fig. 3). They showed a significantly increased Cho/Cr ratio in undifferentiated cancer compared with SCC. Also, there was no Cho or Cr peak detected in most of the benign lymph nodes. Bisdas and colleagues[20] compared the Cho/Cr ratio between metastatic and benign lymph nodes in patients with head and neck cancers and concluded that the Cho/Cr ratio was significantly higher in metastatic lymph nodes.

Prediction of Treatment Outcome

The prediction of treatment outcome is important to optimize individual management such as the selection of treatment regimen or posttreatment follow-up strategy. Several studies were performed to demonstrate the prediction of treatment outcome using MRS. In an early report by Bezabeh and colleagues,[27] various primary sites of HNSCC treated mostly by surgery were analyzed with ex-vivo MRS scanning of a surgical specimen or biopsy fragment. In this study, the Cho/Cr ratio was significantly elevated in the local failure group compared with the local control group. In addition, spectral intensity ratio of 1.3/0.9 ppm (explained as lipid or lactate concentration) was significantly elevated in the local failure group. The best diagnostic accuracy was obtained using 1.3/0.9 ppm ratio noting sensitivity of 83% and specificity of 82%. In contrast, Le and colleagues[28] described that the Cho/Cr ratio and lactate concentration within metastatic lymph nodes was not significantly correlated to treatment outcome in patients who received chemoradiation therapy. King and colleagues[29] evaluated the utility of Cho/Cr ratios in patients with HNSCC who underwent definitive chemoradiotherapy/radiotherapy by placing the VOI in their primary site; however, neither pre- nor intratreatment Cho/Cr ratios correlated with prognosis. The reasons for these contradictory results are still unclear. One could wonder whether the differences in treatment might have affected the results because patients in Le and colleagues' study were treated with surgery and patients in King and colleagues' study were treated with chemoradiation. Moreover, the differences among MR equipment, scan parameters, and distribution of primary tumor site could be factors contributing to varied study results. Recently, pretreatment evaluation with the combination of the ^{1}H-MRS and fluorodeoxyglucose PET (FDG-PET) parameters was reported.[30] In this study, Kaplan-Meier analysis identified two ^{1}H-MRS parameters—lower Cr level and higher glutamine and glutamate (Glx) level (2.2–2.4 ppm)—to be significant predictors for 2-year local failure in

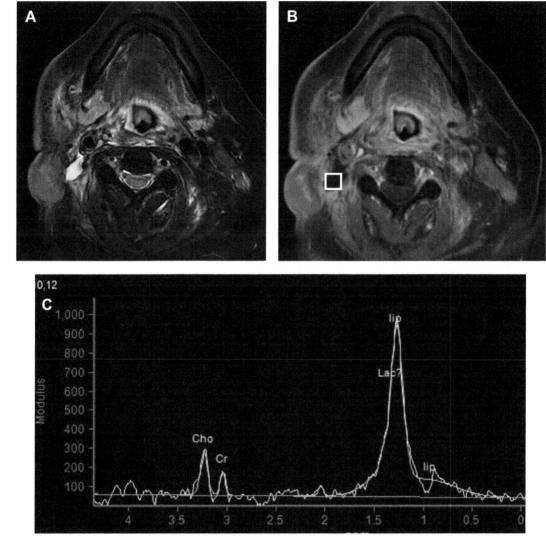

Fig. 3. ¹H-MRS in a necrotic recurrent SCC. Axial T2-weighted (A) and postcontrast T1-weighted (B) images in a 66-year-old man with a history of treated laryngeal cavity SCC demonstrates a centrally necrotic enhancing mass in the right neck with adjacent skin extension that was pathologically proven to be a lymph nodal recurrence with extranodal extension. A VOI has been placed over the nonenhancing necrotic portion. The corresponding ¹H-MRS spectrum (C) shows an elevated peak around 1.3 ppm, likely representative of a combination of lipid and lactate peaks, both of which have been observed in necrotic tumors. This spectrum also illustrates the difficulty in separating lipid and lactate peaks that can significantly overlap at this level and hence is marked lip/lac by the automated algorithm.

patients with HNSCC who received chemoradiation therapy. In addition, multivariate Cox regression analysis revealed Glx was an independent predictor of treatment outcome as well as total lesion glycolysis obtained by FDG-PET. Cho level was not significant as a predictor of treatment outcome in this report.

To date, there have been very few studies investigating the predictive power of MRS in the setting of head and neck cancer. Further investigation is needed to determine the utility of MRS parameters for treatment outcome and prognosis prediction.

Posttreatment Prediction of Residual or Recurrent Tumor

In 2007, Bisdas and colleagues[20] reported MRS may be useful to assess the presence of residual tumor after chemotherapy. In their study, 8 patients with posttreatment granulation tissue without residual tumor showed lower Cho peaks relative to surrounding normal tissue, whereas 3 recurrent tumors showed elevated Cho peaks. However, Cho peak elevation was not identified in 2 patients with recurrent tumors. In another study by King and colleagues[29] published in 2010, several patients (4/9) with posttreatment granulation with residual cancer tissue showed elevated Cho/Cr ratio, whereas none of the patients with posttreatment granulation without residual cancer (0/21) showed elevation of Cho/Cr ratio. They concluded that the presence of a Cho peak was useful to detect residual tumor with high specificity (100%). Based on these 2 studies, the presence of an elevated Cho peak in posttreatment tissue suggests residual or recurrent tumor with high specificity; however, the absence of an elevated Cho peak does not exclude residual or recurrent tumor.

Correlation of Magnetic Resonance Spectroscopy Parameters with Other Modalities and Parameters

Some investigators performed correlational studies between MRS derived parameters and parameters derived from other imaging modalities or histologic findings.

Jansen and colleagues reported that Cho concentration (Cho/water ratio) showed a significant positive correlation to FDG-PET derived total lesion glycolysis (r = 0.599).[31] They discussed high Cho/water ratio indicates increased membrane turnover, which suggests high cellular proliferation, whereas increased glucose metabolism is also related to increased cellular proliferation. In the same study, perfusion-derived parameters obtained from dynamic contrast-enhanced (DCE) MR were evaluated. A significant negative correlation to standard deviation of v_e (mean volume fraction of the extravascular extracellular space [EES]) (r = −0.69) and of k_{ep} (mean rate constant between plasma and EES) (r = −0.7) were reported. Heterogeneity of DCE perfusion parameters and Cho elevation is somewhat difficult to interpret; however, they discussed that heterogeneous areas in tumors often contain highly necrotic regions, which appear as low cellular proliferation due to the presence of necrosis.

In comparison to histopathological parameters, Jansen and colleagues[32] reported that Cho concentration (Cho/water ratio) showed moderate correlation (r = 0.597) to histopathological Ki-67 index (a nuclear marker of cellular proliferation measured by immunohistochemistry), although statistical significance was not observed. This study was performed with a very small number of subjects (n = 12); it is possible that statistical significance could be reached with a larger sample size analysis. A study by Matsumura and colleagues[33] demonstrated a positive correlation between Cho/Cr ratio and Ki-67 index in brain tumors. Head and neck tumors may demonstrate a similar tendency. Another study by Tse and colleagues[34] showed correlation of MRS-derived parameters and several tumor biological markers obtained histologically. In this study, Cho/Cr ratio demonstrated correlation to cyclooxygenase 2 (COX-2) in the primary tumor and epidermal growth factor (EGFR) receptor in metastatic cervical lymph nodes (r = 0.714 and 0.522, respectively). In a more recent study published in 2016, the correlation analysis of Cho/Cr ratio and apparent diffusion coefficient value derived from diffusion-weighted imaging was performed.[35] A significant negative correlation was observed between these 2 parameters. In addition, Cho/Cr ratio in well- or moderately differentiated SCC was significantly lower than in poorly differentiated SCC or undifferentiated cancer.

According to these studies, evaluation of MRS parameters, especially Cho elevation, may have clinical value as indicators for the noninvasive assessment of tumor biological profile.

Chemical Shift Imaging

Most MRS investigations in the head and neck were achieved using single voxel technique. Multivoxel imaging is still challenging in the head and neck, mainly because it needs too long an acquisition time and high-quality shimming in a wide range. In a study that evaluated the feasibility of CSI, the investigators tried to improve the acquisition conditions at 3.0 T field strength by using second-order shimming with perfluorocarbon pads around the neck.[36] Among 14 patients, CSI was successfully obtained in 10 patients with nodal metastases (n = 8) and benign tumors (n = 2), although it was unsuccessful in 4 patients with primary tumors of the aerodigestive tract.

^{31}P-MRS: PRINCIPLE AND CLINICAL UTILITY

^{31}P-MRS is a noninvasive technique that can provide information about energy and phospholipid metabolism. The ^{31}P-MRS spectrum provides various signals from phosphomonoesters (PMEs; phospholipid precursors) and phosphodiesters (PDEs; phospholipid catabolites), inorganic phosphate (Pi), phosphocreatine (PCr), and nucleotide triphosphates (NTPs) related to energy metabolism. This technique has been widely used in the evaluation of muscle metabolism,[37] and there

have been several studies that evaluate head and neck tumors.[38-44]

Acquisition

In the acquisition of ^{31}P-MRS, the chemical-shift imaging sequence with proton decoupling and nuclear Overhauser enhancement with dual-tuned ^{1}H/^{31}P surface coil was reported in 2001.[42] By using this acquisition technique, better localization of the target lesion with further signal increase and well-defined spectral lines can be obtained compared with conventional single-tuned surface coil technique. Other acquisition techniques were mostly similar to that of ^{1}H-MRS. However, because of the relatively poor SNR in ^{31}P-MRS compared with ^{1}H-MRS, the required voxel size tends to be larger (typically larger than 2.0 cm × 2.0 cm × 2.0 cm), and acquisition time becomes longer (around 10–30 min).

Metabolites

The ^{31}P-MRS spectrum includes the following 7 peaks: PME, Pi, PDE, PCr, and 3 nucleotide triphosphates (α-NTP [doublet], β-NTP [doublet], and γ-NTP [triplet]). The NTP includes the signal from adenosine triphosphate, adenosine diphosphate, and adenosine monophosphate. The PME is meant to reflect phospholipid cell membrane precursors and includes signal from phosphocholine, phosphoethanolamine, adenosine monophosphate, and glucose-6-phosphate. The PDE peak reflects cell membrane degradation products, including glycerophosphorylcholine and glycerophosphorylethanolamine. The total phosphorus metabolism is estimated as the sum of the intensities for all peaks (total metabolite signal) in the spectrum except PCr.

Clinical Investigations

According to several investigators, the analysis of ^{31}P-MRS peaks in head and neck tumors has shown elevated levels of PME and PDE in tumors compared with normal neck muscles.[39,44] In addition, HNSCC showed increased levels of Pi, which may be associated with necrosis within the tumors.[2,40] In contrast, decreased levels of PCr in HNSCC were observed compared with normal neck muscles.[40]

Regarding the prediction of treatment outcome in patients with HNSCC, although the pretreatment peaks of PME and PDE were not significantly different between complete remission (CR) and non-CR in patients with HNSCC who had received chemoradiotherapy, marked decreases of both peaks were observed in posttreatment site tissue in the CR group compared with the non-CR group.[40] In contrast, another study reported that in patients with HNSCC treated by chemoradiotherapy, pretreatment PME peaks were significantly lower in the CR group than in the non-CR group. The investigators suggested that the pretreatment PME peak might be a useful predictor of outcome.[41] Only a few studies of ^{31}P-MRS for head and neck lesions have been published, therefore, further studies are desired to confirm these results.

FUTURE PERSPECTIVE

In recent years, the number of clinical studies applying MRS techniques to head and neck lesions has not increased substantially. This might change in the future, with renewed interest due to the increasing availability of high field strength MR units such as 3T or 7T. The use of higher field strengths and application of new high-order shimming techniques may enable higher SNR, more stable spectral baseline, and improved detection and separation of metabolite peaks. These advantages will contribute to evaluation of metabolites in greater detail even with very small single voxels or CSI. As more studies demonstrate the clinical value of MRS for treatment planning and posttreatment monitoring in the head and neck, MRS has the possibility to attract greater attention from head and neck surgeons and oncologists in the near future.

DISCLOSURE

The authors have nothing to disclose.

REFERENCES

1. Srinivasan A, Mohan S, Mukherji SK. Biologic imaging of head and neck cancer: the present and the future. AJNR Am J Neuroradiol 2012;33:586–94.
2. Abdel Razek AA, Poptani H. MR spectroscopy of head and neck cancer. Eur J Radiol 2013;82:982–9.
3. Bhatnagar P, Subesinghe M, Patel C, et al. Functional imaging for radiation treatment planning, response assessment, and adaptive therapy in head and neck cancer. Radiographics 2013;33: 1909–29.
4. King AD, Thoeny HC. Functional MRI for the prediction of treatment response in head and neck squamous cell carcinoma: potential and limitations. Cancer Imaging 2016;16:23.
5. Yuan J, Lo G, King AD. Functional magnetic resonance imaging techniques and their development for radiation therapy planning and monitoring in the head and neck cancers. QuantImaging Med Surg 2016;6:430–48.

6. Dai YL, King AD. State of the art MRI in head and neck cancer. Clin Radiol 2018;73:45–59.

7. Haase A, Frahm J, Hanicke W, et al. ^{1}H NMR chemical shift selective (CHESS) imaging. Phys Med Biol 1985;30:341–4.

8. Mullins ME. MR spectroscopy: truly molecular imaging; past, present and future. Neuroimaging Clin N Am 2006;16:605–18.

9. Delikatny EJ, Chawla S, Leung DJ, et al. MR-visible lipids and the tumor microenvironment. NMR Biomed 2011;24:592–611.

10. Somashekar BS, Kamarajan P, Danciu T, et al. Magic angle spinning NMR-based metabolic profiling of head and neck squamous cell carcinoma tissues. J Proteome Res 2011;10:5232–41.

11. Mukherji SK, Schiro S, Castillo M, et al. Proton MR spectroscopy of squamous cell carcinoma of the upper aerodigestive tract: in vitro characteristics. AJNR Am J Neuroradiol 1996;17:1485–90.

12. Mukherji SK, Schiro S, Castillo M, et al. Proton MR spectroscopy of squamous cell carcinoma of the extracranial head and neck: in vitro and in vivo studies. AJNR Am J Neuroradiol 1997;18:1057–72.

13. Maheshwari SR, Mukherji SK, Neelon B, et al. The choline/creatine ratio in five benign neoplasms: comparison with squamous cell carcinoma by use of in vitro MR spectroscopy. AJNR Am J Neuroradiol 2000;21:1930–5.

14. El-Sayed S, Bezabeh T, Odlum O, et al. An ex vivo study exploring the diagnostic potential of ^{1}H magnetic resonance spectroscopy in squamous cell carcinoma of the head and neck region. Head Neck 2002;24:766–72.

15. King AD, Yeung DK, Ahuja AT, et al. In vivo proton MR spectroscopy of primary and nodal nasopharyngeal carcinoma. AJNR Am J Neuroradiol 2004;25: 484–90.

16. King AD, Yeung DK, Ahuja AT, et al. In vivo ^{1}H MR spectroscopy of thyroid carcinoma. Eur J Radiol 2005;54:112–7.

17. Yu Q, Yang J, Wang P. Malignant tumors and chronic infections in the masticator space: preliminary assessment with in vivo single-voxel [1]H-MR spectroscopy. AJNR Am J Neuroradiol 2008;29:716–9.

18. Yu Q, Yang J, Wang P, et al. Preliminary assessment of benign maxillofacial and neck lesions with in vivo single-voxel ^{1}H magnetic resonance spectroscopy. Oral Surg Oral Med Oral Pathol Oral Radiol Endod 2007;104:264–70.

19. Krouwer HG, Kim TA, Rand SD, et al. Single-voxel proton MR spectroscopy of nonneoplastic brain lesions suggestive of a neoplasm. AJNR Am J Neuroradiol 1998;19:1695–703.

20. Bisdas S, Baghi M, Huebner F, et al. In vivo proton MR spectroscopy of primary tumours, nodal and recurrent disease of the extracranial head and neck. Eur Radiol 2007;17:251–7.

21. King AD, Yeung DK, Ahuja AT, et al. Salivary gland tumors at in vivo proton MR spectroscopy. Radiology 2005;237:563–9.

22. Zhu L, Wang J, Shi H, et al. Multimodality fMRI with perfusion, diffusion-weighted MRI and (1) H-MRS in the diagnosis of lympho-associated benign and malignant lesions of the parotid gland. J Magn Reson Imaging 2019;49:423–32.

23. Gupta N, Kakar AK, Chowdhury V, et al. Magnetic resonance spectroscopy as a diagnostic modality for carcinoma thyroid. Eur J Radiol 2007;64: 414–8.

24. Aydin H, Kizilgoz V, Tatar I, et al. The role of proton MR spectroscopy and apparent diffusion coefficient values in the diagnosis of malignant thyroid nodules: preliminary results. Clin Imaging 2012; 36:323–33.

25. Aghaghazvini L, Pirouzi P, Sharifian H, et al. 3T magnetic resonance spectroscopy as a powerful diagnostic modality for assessment of thyroid nodules. Arch Endocrinol Metab 2018;62:501–5.

26. King AD, Yeung DK, Ahuja AT, et al. Human cervical lymphadenopathy: evaluation with in vivo ^{1}H-MRS at 1.5 T. Clin Radiol 2005;60:592–8.

27. Bezabeh T, Odlum O, Nason R, et al. Prediction of treatment response in head and neck cancer by magnetic resonance spectroscopy. AJNR Am J Neuroradiol 2005;26:2108–13.

28. Le QT, Koong A, Lieskovsky YY, et al. In vivo ^{1}H magnetic resonance spectroscopy of lactate in patients with stage IV head and neck squamous cell carcinoma. Int J Radiat Oncol Biol Phys 2008;71: 1151–7.

29. King AD, Yeung DK, Yu KH, et al. Monitoring of treatment response after chemoradiotherapy for head and neck cancer using in vivo ^{1}H MR spectroscopy. Eur Radiol 2010;20:165–72.

30. Yeh CH, Lin G, Wang JJ, et al. Predictive value of ^{1}H MR spectroscopy and ^{18}F-FDG PET/CT for local control of advanced oropharyngeal and hypopharyngeal squamous cell carcinoma receiving chemoradiotherapy: a prospective study. Oncotarget 2017;8:115513–25.

31. Jansen JF, Schoder H, Lee NY, et al. Tumor metabolism and perfusion in head and neck squamous cell carcinoma: pretreatment multimodality imaging with ^{1}H magnetic resonance spectroscopy, dynamic contrast-enhanced MRI, and [18F]FDG-PET. Int J Radiat Oncol Biol Phys 2012;82:299–307.

32. Jansen JF, Carlson DL, Lu Y, et al. Correlation of a priori DCE-MRI and (1)H-MRS data with molecular markers in neck nodal metastases: Initial analysis. Oral Oncol 2012;48:717–22.

33. Matsumura A, Isobe T, Anno I, et al. Correlation between choline and MIB-1 index in human gliomas. A quantitative in proton MR spectroscopy study. J Clin Neurosci 2005;12:416–20.

34. Tse GM, King AD, Yu AM, et al. Correlation of bio-markers in head and neck squamous cell carcinoma. Otolaryngol HeadNeck Surg 2010;143: 795–800.

35. Razek AA, Nada N. Correlation of choline/creatine and apparent diffusion coefficient values with the prognostic parameters of head and neck squamous cell carcinoma. NMR Biomed 2016;29:483–9.

36. Yeung DK, Fong KY, Chan QC, et al. Chemical shift imaging in the head and neck at 3T: initial results. J Magn Reson Imaging 2010;32:1248–54.

37. Taylor DJ. Clinical utility of muscle MR spectroscopy. Semin Musculoskelet Radiol 2000;4:481–502.

38. McKenna WG, Lenkinski RE, Hendrix RA, et al. The use of magnetic resonance imaging and spectroscopy in the assessment of patients with head and neck and other superficial human malignancies. Cancer 1989;64:2069–75.

39. Vogl T, Peer F, Schedel H, et al. ^{31}P-spectroscopy of head and neck tumors–surface coil technique. Magn Reson Imaging 1989;7:425–35.

40. Maldonado X, Alonso J, Giralt J, et al. [31]Phosphorus magnetic resonance spectroscopy in the assessment of head and neck tumors. Int J Radiat Oncol Biol Phys 1998;40:309–12.

41. Shukla-Dave A, Poptani H, Loevner LA, et al. Prediction of treatment response of head and neck cancers with P-31 MR spectroscopy from pretreatment relative phosphomonoester levels. Acad Radiol 2002;9:688–94.

42. Klomp DW, Collins DJ, van den Boogert HJ, et al. Radio-frequency probe for ^{1}H decoupled ^{31}P MRS of the head and neck region. Magn Reson Imaging 2001;19:755–9.

43. Chawla S, Kim S, Loevner LA, et al. Proton and phosphorous MR spectroscopy in squamous cell carcinomas of the head and neck. Acad Radiol 2009;16:1366–72.

44. Hendrix RA, Lenkinski RE, Vogele K, et al. [31]P localized magnetic resonance spectroscopy of head and neck tumors–preliminary findings. Otolaryngol HeadNeck Surg 1990;103:775–83.

Technical Improvements in Head and Neck MR Imaging
At the Cutting Edge

Gregory Avey, MD*

KEYWORDS

- MR imaging • Head and neck • Dixon • PET/MR imaging • ZTE • Deep learning
- Compressed sensing

KEY POINTS

- MR imaging of the head and neck is becoming more capable and reliable with advancing MR imaging technology.
- Dixon, STIR, and hybrid fat-saturation techniques generate homogenously fat-saturated images over large fields of view despite magnetic field inhomogeneity.
- Diffusion and perfusion/permeability imaging and other functional techniques are becoming more reliable and easier to implement because of novel acquisition strategies.
- Compressed sensing and deep learning reconstruction techniques allow for accelerated image acquisition through limited subsampling of k-space.
- Simultaneous PET/MR imaging allows for an 80% radiation dose reduction and allows advanced tumor characterization through functional imaging techniques.

INTRODUCTION

The anatomy of the head and neck is technically challenging with regard to reliably obtaining high-quality MR images. The structures of clinical interest, such as cranial nerves, are often diminutive in size and require high-resolution imaging.[1] Variation in cross-sectional diameter through the neck causes challenges in MR imaging coil design and also results in magnetic field inhomogeneity. Magnetic field inhomogeneity is also common about the orbit and temporal bone because of air-tissue interfaces, compromising the image quality of conventional MR imaging sequences.[2,3] Motion from swallowing and respiration can compromise imaging throughout the neck and particularly at the thoracic inlet. In response to these challenges MR imaging technology has advanced with improvements in coil construction, MR imaging sequence design, fat saturation techniques, and the advent of innovative acceleration techniques.

These technical advances have alleviated many of the challenges of head and neck MR imaging, allowing the clinician to leverage the many advantages of MR imaging including improved tissue contrast compared with computed tomography (CT), the lack of ionizing radiation, and the addition of functional imaging sequences. This results in improved diagnostic and prognostic specificity. MR imaging in the head and neck has been paired with simultaneous PET, increasing the opportunities for functional imaging of the head and neck. These advances allow for more accurate diagnosis and staging of head and neck tumors, and promises to allow for more individualized therapy based on prognostic imaging markers. This review focuses on cutting-edge technical improvements in head and neck MR imaging to allow readers to optimize their current head and neck protocols and serves as a review to highlight advances just moving into clinical practice.

Radiology, University of Wisconsin, Madison, WI, USA
* 600 Highland Avenue, Madison, WI 53792.
E-mail address: gavey@uwhealth.org

Neuroimag Clin N Am 30 (2020) 295–309
https://doi.org/10.1016/j.nic.2020.04.002

neuroimaging.theclinics.com

ADVANCES IN MORPHOLOGIC SEQUENCES

Given the anatomic complexity and need to assess for perineural tumor spread, an image thickness less than 3 mm is recommended within the head and neck.[1] Imaging of the temporal bone, orbit, and cerebellopontine angle may require even thinner and higher resolution images for adequate evaluation.[4] Generation of thin two-dimensional (2D) images with conventional techniques is time intensive, creating a tension between the need for thin images and time efficient MR imaging protocols. There have been advances in fast spin echo (FSE) and gradient echo–based sequences, which allow the generation of thin isovolumetric three-dimensional (3D) data sets in times that are comparable with conventional 2D based techniques, but with much thinner slice width.[5] These sequences have the additional advantage of allowing reformatting in any user-defined plane. This can eliminate the need for one or more standard 2D acquisitions, decreasing overall MR imaging examination times.[6] The isovolumetric nature of these examinations also supports the 3D needs of those planning and implementing radiation therapy.[7]

Three-Dimensional Fast Spin Echo–Based Techniques

Because of the presence of refocusing pulses, FSE-based techniques are less susceptible to magnetic field inhomogeneity. However, conventional FSE-based imaging pulses using full 180° refocusing pulses have limited useable echo train lengths, increased energy deposition/specific absorption rate (SAR), and result in image blurring. With variable flip angles of less than 180° in magnitude, long echo train lengths can be used on the order of 100 to 250 echoes per TR.[5] 3D pulse sequences using these techniques, such as SPACE, CUBE, or VISTA, are combined with parallel imaging and acceleration techniques to allow for millimeter or submillimeter imaging encompassing large fields of view in clinically acceptable imaging times.[8] Most common tissue weightings are available with these sequences, including T1, T2, proton density (PD), fluid-attenuated inversion recovery (FLAIR), short tau inversion recovery (STIR), and double inversion recovery (DIR). These techniques can also be paired with black blood imaging techniques and robust Dixon-based fat-saturation to provide images with robust fat saturation and decreased pulsation artifact.[9]

Three-Dimensional MR Imaging Cisternography

Heavily T2-weighted sequences are frequently used in head and neck MR imaging to evaluate the cisternal segments of cranial nerves and the fluid-filled labyrinth of the inner ear. Conventionally, balanced steady-state free precession (bSSFP)-based sequences have been used for this task (FIESTA, CISS, TrueFISP).[7] These gradient echo–based sequences have a signal intensity of T2/T1, with the high T2 signal intensity of cerebrospinal fluid resulting in the characteristic intracranial cisternogram/hyperintense cerebrospinal fluid appearance.[10] This unusual tissue contrast characteristic (T2/T1) also results in an increased signal intensity within vascular structures, such as the cavernous sinus and jugular foramen following the administration of gadolinium-based contrast agents. This enables evaluation of these cranial nerve branches as they transit these vascular structures, extending the diagnostic reach of this form of MR imaging cisternogram imaging.[11,12] Unfortunately, these sequences are also prone to MR imaging banding artifacts arising from areas of magnetic inhomogeneity. These banding artifacts are decreased by performing two acquisitions with differing phase directions, but are often not completely eliminated.[10]

Heavily T2-weighted 3D FSE-based sequences (SPACE, CUBE, VISTA) have more recently been applied to MR imaging cisternography. These sequences do not suffer from the banding artifacts of bSSFP images, but also lack the advantageous contrast enhancement characteristics of the bSSFP sequences. 3D FSE-based techniques have been shown to have greater contrast to noise compared with bSSFP images, and suffer from fewer susceptibility and vascular flow-related artifacts.[13,14] Additionally, 3D FSE-based images demonstrate improved visualization of the entire length of the cisternal cranial nerves compared with bSSFP-based images.[15]

Three-Dimensional Fluid-Attenuated Inversion Recovery Applications in the Head and Neck

Although conventionally considered a brain imaging sequence, 3D FSE FLAIR has found several significant applications in head and neck imaging. 3D FLAIR is more sensitive to low concentrations of gadolinium-based contrast agents compared with more conventional T1-based tissue contrast techniques.[16] This unusual feature of what is typically considered a T2 contrast-based technique has found application in imaging of endolymphatic hydrops. Although the first descriptions of this technique described intratympanic administration of gadolinium-based contrast agents, more recent protocols have transitioned to a delayed imaging protocol, with imaging commencing 4 hours after the intravenous administration of contrast.[17,18] Gadolinium-based contrast slowly accumulates within the perilymph, with dilated endolymphatic structures identified as filling defects within the enhancing perilymph.[19]

3D FLAIR imaging has also been found to be predictive in cases of sudden sensorineural hearing loss, with increased FLAIR signal intensity correlating with more severe hearing loss and poor hearing outcomes (**Fig. 1**).[20–22] In orbit imaging FLAIR hyperintensity of the optic nerve head on contrast-enhanced 3D FLAIR has been shown to closely correlate with the physical examination finding of papilledema in patients with idiopathic intracranial hypertension.[23]

Three-Dimensional Contrast-Enhanced Spoiled Gradient Echo Sequences

In addition to the FSE based techniques described previously, fast gradient echo techniques should also be considered when designing head and neck MR imaging protocols (**Fig. 2**). These sequences (VIBE, LAVA, THRIVE) are performed with accelerated sampling of k-space and paired with robust Dixon-based fat saturation techniques (described later). These techniques have been extensively used in abdominal imaging, and have been designed to allow imaging of the liver

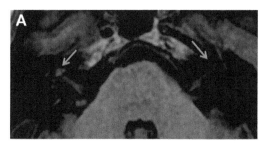

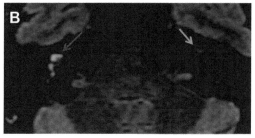

Fig. 1. Patient with sudden sensorineural hearing loss. (*A*) There is no difference in T1 signal intensity (*green arrows*). (*B*) However, there is increased postcontrast FLAIR signal intensity within the right cochlea and labyrinth, suggesting a poor prognosis with respect to hearing outcome (*red arrow, normal side blue arrow*).

parenchyma over a 15- to 20-second (or less) sampling window.[24] When used in the neck at sufficient resolution, typical sequence times are on the order of 2 to 3 minutes. When evaluated in the head and neck, these sequences have been shown to have improved overall image quality and fat suppression compared with conventional FSE-based images, with less respiratory and pulsation artifact.[25] However, the conspicuity of gadolinium-based contrast enhancement may be reduced for these gradient echo–based images as compared with FSE-based sequences.[26]

Zero TE/Black Bone Imaging

There is ongoing interest in substituting ionizing radiation-free MR imaging for CT as part of the effort to limit the radiation exposure because of medical imaging.[27,28] However, the lack of visualization of cortical bone on MR imaging has been one limit to direct substitution, particularly when evaluating for craniosynostosis, fracture, and dysplasia of the midface and mandible. In black bone or zero TE imaging there is little or no delay between the excitation radio frequency (RF) pulse and the implementation of the read-out gradients. This allows for imaging of tissues with short T2 characteristics, such as tendons, menisci, cartilage, and cortical bone.[29] Additionally, this technique is commonly implemented using continuously varying gradients, small flip angles, and a radial sampling of k-space. This creates a near silent scan with imaging times of 2 to 3 minutes for published protocols.[30] The resulting raw image renders cortical bone as low in signal intensity compared with adjacent soft tissues. To create images more comparable with CT, these images undergo a logarithmic inversion and a histogram-based subtraction of air-containing structures. The resulting images have been used for radiation therapy planning and for attenuation correction for PET/MR imaging.[31] There has been reported success with using zero TE images to characterize craniosynostosis along with a variety of developmental and acquired malformations of the calvarium, midface, and mandible.[32,33] However, the sensitivity of current implementations is less than that of CT for nondisplaced linear calvarial fractures and fractures of aerated bone, and therefore the current technique is not recommended for replacing CT in trauma imaging.[34,35]

METHODS OF FAT SUPPRESSION

Fat suppression within the neck is advantageous for evaluation for perineural spread of tumor, increasing the conspicuity of nodal metastasis, and helping to better delineate tumors and

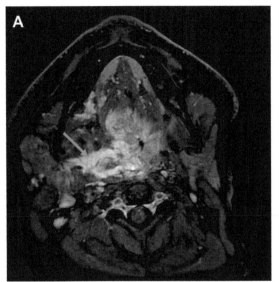
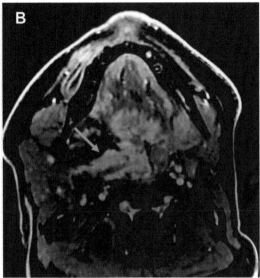

Fig. 2. Patient with venous malformation (*arrow*). Comparison between axial FSE T1 with Dixon fat-saturation (*A*) and reformatted 3D spoiled gradient echo sequence (*B*). Both images demonstrate the full extent of the malformation, with the spoiled gradient echo–based image requiring 2 minutes less imaging time to acquire (4:31 seconds vs 2:30 seconds). The 3D image can effectively replace multiple separately acquired 2D image sequences.

inflammatory processes.[1] However, conventional spectral fat suppression within the neck is commonly compromised by magnetic field inhomogeneity.[36] A variety of techniques have been developed to provide robust fat suppression within the neck with limited time penalty.[37]

STIR is an inversion recovery technique that uses a 180° inversion pulse to null the signal from tissues with a T1 recovery time of fat (approximately 160–180 ms). The resulting images are less reliant on magnetic field homogeneity as compared with spectral fat suppression, at the cost of decreased signal to noise and a slightly increased imaging time. Of note, STIR cannot be used for fat suppression following gadolinium-based contrast administration, because the T1 shortening properties of the contrast agent may place the T1 relaxation rate of tissues of interest into the band nulled by the STIR inversion pulse.[38] As such, STIR is predominately at T2-weighted technique.

There are also hybrid techniques that use a spectrally selective pulse to selectively invert and null the signal from fat, combining elements of spectral and STIR fat suppression. These techniques (SPIR, SPECIAL) may be used for postcontrast T1 images, but are prone to failure in areas of magnetic inhomogeneity.[39,40]

Dixon-based techniques rely on the slight differences in the resonant frequency of protons within water and fat. At 1.5 T, these protons cycle between being in phase and out of phase every 4.4 milliseconds. This allows the generation of "fat only" and "water only" images by imaging at in phase and out of phase time points (**Fig. 3**). This method produces robust fat-water separation that is not dependent on magnetic field homogeneity (**Fig. 4**).[41] This technique is used for T1, T2, and postcontrast imaging, unlike STIR. These methods differ in the number of echoes required to produce the fat-water separation, with three-point Dixon techniques (IDEAL) requiring a longer examination time than two-point techniques (FLEX, mDixon, FatSep). Dixon fat-water separation techniques are applied to 2D and 3D techniques, and are particularly effective in allowing for homogenous fat saturation in the large field of views associated with 3D imaging. Dixon-based fat-water separation techniques have been found to offer better image quality and more uniform fat suppression at lower imaging times when compared with STIR-based techniques.[40]

DIFFUSION WEIGHTING OPTIONS

Diffusion-weighted imaging has a myriad of uses within the head and neck. Diffusion is a highly accurate method of distinguishing between infantile hemangiomas and rhabdomyosarcomas in the pediatric population, differentiating between inflammatory and neoplastic masses within the orbit, and separating cholesteatoma from proteinaceous secretions within the temporal bone (**Fig.

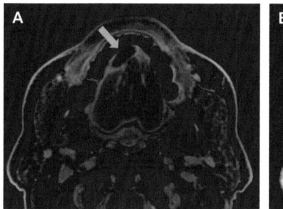
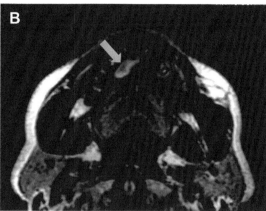

Fig. 3. Water (*A*) and fat (*B*) postcontrast T1-weighted images demonstrating a lesion that is low in signal intensity on the water images. This lesion superficially resembles a ranula on the water images (*blue arrow*), but demonstrates macroscopic fat on the fat-water separation images (*green arrow*). Based on the MR imaging results this lesion was biopsied, and was found to be a spindle cell lipoma on pathologic review.

5).[42–44] Pretreatment diffusion-weighted imaging has also been shown to predict the response of head and neck squamous cell carcinoma to radiation therapy.[45,46] Additionally, lesions that fail to increase in ADC value early in the course of radiation therapy are likely to result in treatment failure.[47,48]

Diffusion-weighted techniques within the head and neck are broadly separated into echo planar imaging (EPI)-based techniques and spin echo–based techniques.[49] The single-shot EPI-based techniques are widely available and are routinely performed as part of brain imaging. These techniques are quickly acquired and as such are

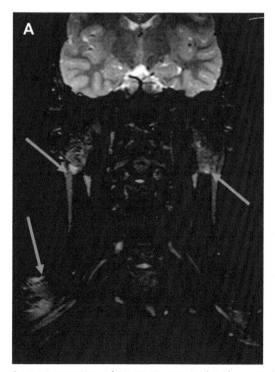
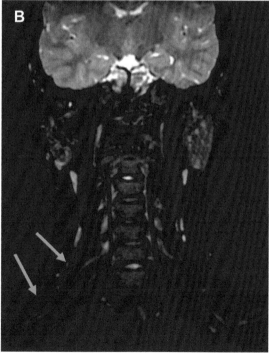

Fig. 4. Comparison of 3D T2 FSE acquired with spectral fat saturation (*A*) and Dixon-based fat-water separation (*B*). There is inhomogeneity of fat saturation with spectral fat saturation (*blue arrows*). The full extent of the brachial plexus is better shown on the Dixon-based image (*green arrows*) because of the homogeneity of fat suppression.

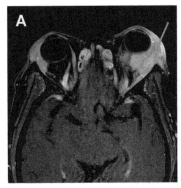
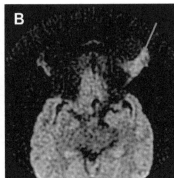
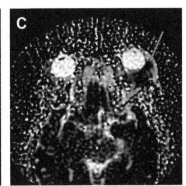

Fig. 5. Postcontrast (*A*), propeller diffusion-weighted (*B*), and ADC (*C*) images of orbital lymphoma (*arrows*) involving the left orbit. Lymphoma typically demonstrates highly restricted diffusion because of its highly cellular nature. Because of magnetic field inhomogeneity, echo planar imaging–based diffusion is not recommended for imaging of the orbit.

motion resistant. However, single-shot EPI diffusion also suffers from limited spatial resolution and susceptibility artifacts, which result in geometric distortion and signal drop out. The segmentation of EPI diffusion over multiple acquisitions significantly reduces the distortion because of magnetic susceptibility, at the penalty of increased examination time. This multishot EPI diffusion is performed at higher resolution than single-shot EPI techniques, and has an overall greater image quality than single-shot techniques in most locations within the head and neck.[50] These techniques should be paired with robust forms of fat suppression, because inhomogeneous suppression of fat on diffusion-weighted imaging can also limit image quality.[50] Limited field-of-view techniques created by selective excitation of the area of interest allows for less distortion and a greater resolution, without the time penalty of multishot EPI diffusion. However, this technique is most applicable for areas of limited tissue volume, such as the sella or spine.[51]

Because of the inherent limitation of EPI-based techniques, FSE-based diffusion-weighted imaging has also been developed. One technique uses a single-shot FSE-based technique to acquire all of the imaging data in one acquisition by having a long echo train.[52,53] Although this imaging technique is rapidly acquired, the single-shot nature and long echo train results in limited resolution and blurring. Multishot FSE techniques are typically sampled as rotating overlapped parallel lines through k-space, limiting susceptibility artifact.[54] However, these FSE techniques come at a significant time penalty compared with EPI-based methods, and are typically reserved for small areas of specific interest, such as the temporal bone when evaluating for cholesteatoma.[55]

Intravoxel incoherent motion (IVIM) is an advanced diffusion imaging method where the diffusion signal from the motion of water molecules within tissue is distinguished from the motion caused by the perfusion of the tissue through the capillary bed. At lower b values (0–200 s/mm^2) the measured b value is a combination of conventional tissue perfusion and water diffusion, whereas at higher b values (400 to >1000 s/mm^2) the contribution from tissue perfusion is negligible. Through measuring multiple b values these components are separated. IVIM typically yields three parameters: D, D*, and f. D represents conventional tissue diffusion, D* the pseudodiffusion component attributable to perfusion, and f the perfusion fraction correlating to the density of capillaries in the tissue being imaged.[56] This creates a single technique through which one can measure diffusion and a marker of tissue perfusion, with early studies suggesting the potential for use in distinguishing benign lymph nodes from lymph nodes harboring metastatic disease.[57]

VASCULAR AND PERFUSION/PERMEABILITY MR IMAGING

The lack of ionizing radiation associated with MR imaging creates the opportunity for rapid sequential imaging, and as such is the modality of choice for techniques evaluating the contrast enhancement characteristics of tissues of the neck and perfusion imaging. These techniques can range from a qualitative assessment of enhancement obtained through repeated conventional images to dedicated time-resolved imaging and formal perfusion MR imaging. These techniques are highly specific in characterization of venous malformations of the orbit and paragangliomas of the skull base from other morphologic similar tumors.[58,59]

Time-resolved imaging techniques are also critical in evaluating vascular lesions of the head and neck.[60,61] Perfusion imaging is useful in evaluating for cervical lymph node metastasis and in predicting tumor response to therapy.[62]

Time-Resolved MR Angiography

Time-resolved MR angiography was initially conceived as a method to more optimally time the arterial arrival of the contrast bolus for MR angiography.[63] However, when performed for greater durations this technique can assess the overall vascularity of tissues, including the phase of peak enhancement and the homogeneity of contrast enhancement. These features are central to the accurate and specific identification of vascular malformations and hypervascular tumors (Fig. 6).[60,61,64] These techniques (TRICKS, TWIST, 4D-TRACK) use a variation on the keyhole method of MR angiography, with more frequent imaging of the center of k-space than the periphery, allowing more frequent imaging of the dominant components of the image while still capturing high resolution and vascular detail. Other work has evaluated the contrast kinetics of lymph node metastasis in cases of head and neck cancer, demonstrating that these lymph nodes demonstrate delayed enhancement, lower peak enhancement, and slower wash-out compared with normal lymph nodes.[65]

Dynamic Contrast Enhancement Perfusion/ Permeability Imaging

Perfusion imaging is a more quantitative method of characterizing the passage of contrast through tissues of interest. This is most commonly implemented through dynamic contrast enhancement (DCE) perfusion in the head and neck, in which change in T1 signal intensity is sequentially measured in tissues of interest after the administration of an MR imaging contrast agent.[66] DCE perfusion is frequently performed for brain

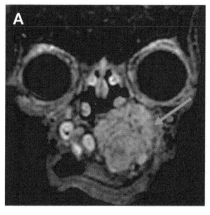

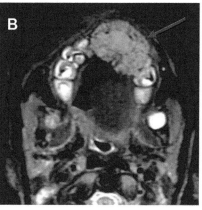

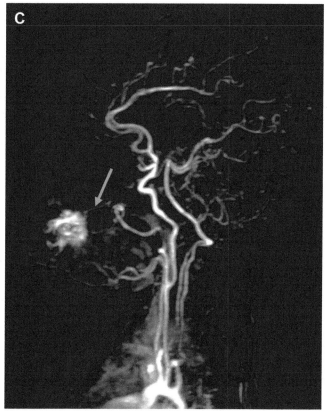

Fig. 6. A highly vascular maxillary mass (*blue and red arrows*) on T1 postcontrast (*A*) and T2-weighted (*B*) images present at birth in this 2-week-old infant with failure to thrive because of the mass interfering with breastfeeding. Time-resolved MR angiography (*C*) demonstrates the early arterial blush of this congenital hemangioma, along with the dominant arterial supply from the greater palatine artery (*green arrow*). This artery was ligated before resection, allowing for safe debulking of the tumor with minimal blood loss.

studies to quantify blood flow changes associated with stroke and treatment-related changes in glioblastoma imaging. DCE perfusion in the head and neck is slightly different than the similar brain study. In the tissues of the head and neck the exchange of molecules is more dynamic than in the brain, because in the brain the blood-brain barrier limits egress of most large molecules (including contrast). In tissues outside of the brain there is a freer exchange of macromolecules and a different model must be used to characterize the exchange in these tissues. The more specific term for characterizing the exchange of molecules in these tissues without a blood tissue barrier is "permeability imaging." Commonly reported markers include capillary permeability, blood volume, blood flow, and mean transit time.[62] These biomarkers show promise in better delineating the extent of head and neck tumor, identification of cervical lymph nodes, prediction of response to therapy, and differentiating recurrent tumor from post-therapeutic changes.[62,67]

There have been notable efforts to improve the standardization of perfusion imaging, with release of recommendations from the Quantitative Imaging Biomarkers Alliance.[68] Key recommendations for the head and neck include precontrast T1 mapping, a temporal resolution of less than 6 seconds, and a total acquisition time of approximately 5 minutes. Commonly used sequences for DCE perfusion include an improved variant of time-resolved MR angiography; differential subsampling with Cartesian ordering; and a radial sampling technique, golden-angle radial sparse parallel imaging.[69–71] These techniques are commonly paired with a fast Dixon-based fat-water separation, allowing for robust fat-water separation along with a rapid sampling interval.

Arterial Spin Labeling Perfusion

As an alternative to DCE perfusion, arterial spin labeling (ASL) perfusion can also be performed in the head and neck. This technique has the advantage of not requiring the injection of a contrast medium. In this method flowing blood is labeled in a tagging zone before flowing into the tissues of interest. The tagged blood then flows into the area of interest, changing the measured signal intensity proportional to the rate of blood flow (**Fig. 7**).[72] The signal-to-noise ratio for ASL perfusion is often low and requires attention to acquisition technique to achieve meaningful images. ASL perfusion has been used in the head and neck to diagnose paragangliomas and differentiate Warthin tumors from pleomorphic adenomas.[73,74] ASL perfusion has also been used to predict treatment response in head and neck tumors, and separate tumor recurrence from post-treatment change.[75,76]

ACCELERATED MR IMAGING
Parallel Imaging

Parallel imaging is an integral part of MR imaging acceleration, and is often combined with the novel techniques described subsequently. There are multiple implementations of this method, but all of these techniques involve the deliberate undersampling of k-space and image acquisition using multiple independent receiver coils, each of which images the anatomy of interest from a unique spatial location. The resulting images are then reconstructed using data regarding individual coil sensitivities to unwrap the individual images into a single large field of view image.[8] The signal to noise in the resulting image is decreased in proportion to the square root of the acceleration factor (ie, for an acceleration factor of 4, the noise is increased by a factor of 2). Residual aliasing in

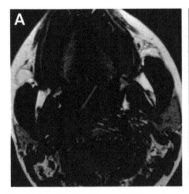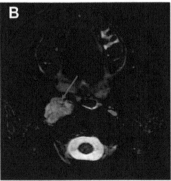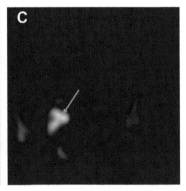

Fig. 7. T1 (*A*), T2 (*B*), and ASL perfusion (*C*) images of a highly vascular skull base mass (*arrows*) discovered during the first trimester of pregnancy. The ASL perfusion images confirmed increased blood flow to this mass, which along with the infiltrative nature of this mass on other images led to a biopsy of this round cell sarcoma.

the image can result in artifacts, which may mimic pathology or mask the underlying anatomy.[77]

Radial/Spiral Acquisition Techniques

A variety of novel k-space acquisition strategies have been created to allow for more rapid image generation. These techniques commonly focus on deliberate undersampling of the periphery of k-space (containing the high frequency "edge" data), and multiple samples of the center of k-space (containing the low-frequency data that make up the main image contrast). These techniques allow for motion correction and faster image acquisition. MR imaging in the head and neck is challenged by respiratory and swallowing artifacts, which propagate in the phase direction as "phase ghost" artifacts. In the head and neck, these artifacts are commonly most significant at the thoracic inlet, limiting evaluation in this region. Non-Cartesian radial and spiral acquisition techniques have been created that help to alleviate these artifacts.[35,71] Because these sequences do not have the traditional separate frequency and phase-encoding directions, patient motion is distributed across the entire image data set instead of propagating in a single direction. The redundant data acquired through each acquisition transitioning through the center of k-space can also be used for motion correction. These sequences have been found to have higher overall image quality and a marked reduction in motion artifacts when compared with conventional sequences.[25,78]

Compressed Sensing

Most of these advanced accelerated imaging techniques rely on the use of undersampling of k-space. On its own, this undersampling can result in poor signal to noise, low resolution, or blurring. Compressed sensing is a technique that is designed to use this undersampling of data points to maximum advantage. Compressed sensing is based on the observation that many MR images are expressed with high fidelity through few data points because of either an intrinsically sparse image (eg, MR angiography), or are able to be represented with few data points after a mathematical transformation because of underlying patterns in the image.[79] Compressed sensing requires three fundamental components. The first, already described, is that the image must be sparse in either the pixel representation or after undergoing an image transform. The second is that there must be either a random or pseudorandom subsampling of data points such that there is no additive effect of image artifacts based on the sampling pattern. Although this is difficult to fully achieve in practice because of the physical limitations in MR imaging hardware, this requirement is well approximated by radial or spiral sampling algorithms. The third component is an iterative reconstruction algorithm that aims to eliminate the noise caused by the pseudorandom sampling while maintaining the integrity to the sampled data points. Compressed sensing is most beneficial for images that are inherently sparse, with MR angiography being an excellent example of a sparse image. Compressed sensing MR angiography allows for similar or improved image quality with a 50% reduction in acquisition time.[80] Other groups have found that compressed sensing allowed an 80% reduction in scan time when screening for vestibular schwannomas while preserving tumor detection rates.[81] Evaluation more broadly has suggested that compressed sensing can achieve a 30% to 60% reduction in imaging time across multiple organ areas without significant degradation in image quality.[82] The three techniques described in this subsection (parallel imaging, radial/spiral acquisition, and compressed sensing) have been combined to allow for improved imaging of parotid and pituitary masses.[83,84]

PET/MR IMAGING

PET/MR imaging is an innovative modality in which solid-state PET detectors are used in conjunction with MR imaging–related attenuation correction to enable simultaneous PET/MR imaging.[85] Attenuation correction of soft tissues for the purposes of accurate PET imaging is achieved through the use of Dixon-based fat-water separation, whereas attenuation correction of osseous structures is typically achieved through the use of short/zero TE images, atlas-based techniques, or transformation of MR images into pseudo-CT images though the use of machine learning algorithms.[86] The solid-state detectors associated with PET/MR imaging are more sensitive than traditional photomultiplier tube–based systems, reducing the PET radiotracer dose required for diagnostic quality images. This reduced PET radiotracer dose, along with elimination of the CT dose component, allows for an up to 80% reduction in the dose of ionizing radiation.[87] This degree of radiation dose decrease is of particular interest in pediatric patients and young patients with head and neck malignancies who may be treated primarily with surgical resection.

The combination of PET and MR imaging into a single examination is useful for patient convenience and has been demonstrated to perform at

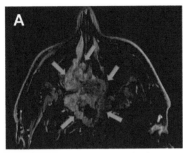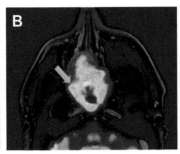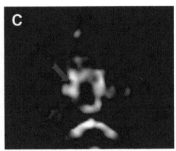

Fig. 8. PET/MR imaging images of an infiltrative mass within the nasopharynx. T1 postcontrast images (*A*) demonstrate an aggressive-appearing mass with extension into the posterior nasal cavity and right maxilla (*blue arrows*). Fluorodeoxyglucose/MR imaging fusion (*B*) demonstrates increased metabolism (*green arrow*) at the periphery of the mass, correlating well with the areas of increased blood flow shown on ASL perfusion (*C*). Of note, the center of the mass is necrotic on imaging with poor blood flow on ASL perfusion (*red arrow*), suggesting a degree of central tumor hypoxia.

least equivalently to PET/CT in the diagnosis and staging of head and neck cancer.[88] The additive advantage of PET/MR imaging is found in combining the morphologic and diagnostic qualities of PET and MR imaging with the functional imaging features discussed previously in this article. In particular, diffusion-weighted imaging, IVIM, and perfusion/permeability MR imaging show promise in predicting tumor response before therapy and within the early stages of therapy (Fig. 8).[62,66,67,69] Similarly, PET activity before therapy and following 2 weeks of chemotherapy and radiation is able to separate early disease responders from those at risk of recurrence.[62,89–92] Following therapy, PET and the functional

components of MR imaging have additive value in assessing for disease recurrence.[93] The predictive value of PET and MR imaging may allow for a greater individualization of therapy, with dose de-escalation and decreased morbidity for early treatment responders.

ARTIFICIAL INTELLIGENCE/DEEP LEARNING RECONSTRUCTION

Conventional MR imaging relies on the use of the inverse Fourier transform to convert the phase and frequency information found in k-space into a diagnostic image.[94] Acceleration in MR imaging often focuses on obtaining only a subset of the

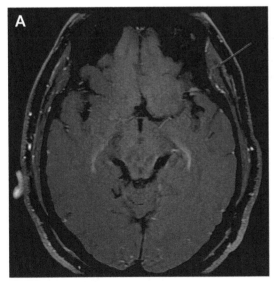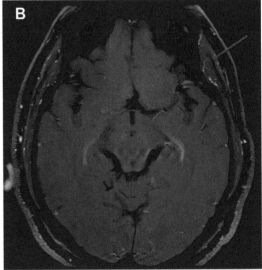

Fig. 9. Conventional (*A*) and deep learning (*B*) reconstructions of a postcontrast T1-weighted image. The deep learning reconstruction has improved signal to noise and improved resolution as demonstrated by improved visualization of small branches of the superficial temporal artery (*red arrows*).

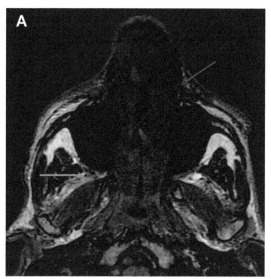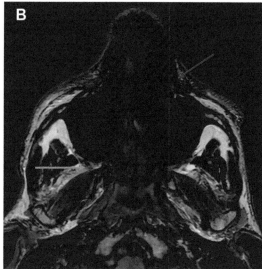

Fig. 10. Conventional (*A*) and deep learning (*B*) reconstructions of a T1-weighted image in a patient with nasal natural killer/T-cell lymphoma with extension into the muscles of facial expression (*red arrows*). There is marked improvement in signal to noise, and improved visualization of the fat within the pterygopalatine fossa (*blue arrows*) on the deep learning reconstructed images.

entirety of k-space data, because obtaining a full representation is time inefficient. However, reconstruction of these sparse data can result in low resolution, blurring, or other data artifacts. Compressed sensing, described previously, has been advanced as one way of extracting high-quality images from these undersampled data sets. Other efforts have turned toward leveraging artificial intelligence/neural networks to reconstruct the limited k-space data (**Figs. 9** and **10**). These approaches have shown promise in accelerating image acquisition, reducing image artifacts, improving signal to noise, and creating "super-resolution" images.[95–98] Depending on the implementation, these techniques are reconstructed in similar or less time than comparable algorithms.[99] The potential for improved acquisition speed is significant, with similar imaging quality resulting from fully sampled images and images with only 25% to 29% of k-space data points sampled.[96] Many of these techniques are agnostic to the underlying imaging sequence, and could be paired with many of the cutting edge techniques previously described to create motion- and artifact-resistant neck MR imaging with uniformly high image quality, along with robust functional techniques in clinically acceptable examination times.[99] These techniques have only recently been described in the literature as regards their use in MR imaging, and many more applications of this technology in image acquisition and reconstruction are anticipated in the near future.

SUMMARY

There have been rapid advancements in MR imaging of the head and neck, with the addition of new morphologic sequences, 3D imaging techniques, robust and time efficient methods of fat saturation, and improved vascular imaging techniques. Developments in functional imaging have also been significant, including advanced methods of permeability imaging, diffusion imaging, and the application of IVIM to the head and neck. The efficient use of these techniques requires the application of accelerated MR imaging methods to reach their full potential, including parallel imaging, novel k-space sampling methods, compressed sensing, and deep learning. These disparate techniques are additive in their impact and show promise in increasing the diagnostic and prognostic capabilities of MR imaging of the head and neck.

REFERENCES

1. Kirsch CFE, Schmalfuss IM. Practical tips for MR imaging of perineural tumor spread. Magn Reson Imaging Clin N Am 2018;26(1):85–100.
2. Herrick RC, Hayman LA, Taber KH, et al. Artifacts and pitfalls in MR imaging of the orbit: a clinical review. Radiographics 1997;17(3):707–24.
3. Oehler MC, Schmalbrock P, Chakeres D, et al. Magnetic susceptibility artifacts on high-resolution MR of the temporal bone. AJNR Am J Neuroradiol 1995; 16(5):1135–43.

4. Glastonbury CM, Davidson HC, Harnsberger HR, et al. Imaging findings of cochlear nerve deficiency. AJNR Am J Neuroradiol 2002;23(4):635–43.

5. Mugler JP 3rd. Optimized three-dimensional fast-spin-echo MRI. J Magn Reson Imaging 2014;39(4): 745–67.

6. Tagliafico A, Succio G, Neumaier CE, et al. Brachial plexus assessment with three-dimensional isotropic resolution fast spin echo MRI: comparison with conventional MRI at 3.0 T. Br J Radiol 2012;85(1014): e110–6.

7. Chandarana H, Wang H, Tijssen RHN, et al. Emerging role of MRI in radiation therapy. J Magn Reson Imaging 2018;48(6):1468–78.

8. Deshmane A, Gulani V, Griswold MA, et al. Parallel MR imaging. J Magn Reson Imaging 2012;36(1): 55–72.

9. Wang D, Lu Y, Yin B, et al. 3D fast spin-echo T1 black-blood imaging for the preoperative detection of venous sinus invasion by meningioma: comparison with contrast-enhanced MRV. Clin Neuroradiol 2019;29(1):65–73.

10. Bieri O, Scheffler K. Fundamentals of balanced steady state free precession MRI. J Magn Reson Imaging 2013;38(1):2–11.

11. Yousry I, Moriggl B, Schmid UD, et al. Trigeminal ganglion and its divisions: detailed anatomic MR imaging with contrast-enhanced 3D constructive interference in the steady state sequences. AJNR Am J Neuroradiol 2005;26(5):1128–35.

12. Linn J, Peters F, Moriggl B, et al. The jugular foramen: imaging strategy and detailed anatomy at 3T. AJNR Am J Neuroradiol 2009;30(1):34–41.

13. Kojima S, Suzuki K, Hirata M, et al. Depicting the semicircular canals with inner-ear MRI: a comparison of the SPACE and TrueFISP sequences. J Magn Reson Imaging 2013;37(3):652–9.

14. Tong T, Yue W, Zhong Y, et al. Comparison of contrast-enhanced SPACE and CISS in evaluating cavernous sinus invasion by pituitary macroadenomas on 3-T magnetic resonance. J Comput Assist Tomogr 2015;39(2):222–7.

15. Ors S, Inci E, Turkay R, et al. Retrospective comparison of three-dimensional imaging sequences in the visualization of posterior fossa cranial nerves. Eur J Radiol 2017;97:65–70.

16. Naganawa S, Kawai H, Sone M, et al. Increased sensitivity to low concentration gadolinium contrast by optimized heavily T2-weighted 3D-FLAIR to visualize endolymphatic space. Magn Reson Med Sci 2010;9(2):73–80.

17. Naganawa S, Yamazaki M, Kawai H, et al. Visualization of endolymphatic hydrops in Meniere's disease with single-dose intravenous gadolinium-based contrast media using heavily T(2)-weighted 3D-FLAIR. Magn Reson Med Sci 2010; 9(4):237–42.

18. van Steekelenburg JM, van Weijnen A, de Pont LMH, et al. Value of endolymphatic hydrops and perilymph signal intensity in suspected Meniere disease. AJNR Am J Neuroradiol 2020;41(3): 529–34.

19. Barath K, Schuknecht B, Naldi AM, et al. Detection and grading of endolymphatic hydrops in Meniere disease using MR imaging. AJNR Am J Neuroradiol 2014;35(7):1387–92.

20. Conte G, Di Berardino F, Sina C, et al. MR imaging in sudden sensorineural hearing loss. Time to talk. AJNR Am J Neuroradiol 2017;38(8):1475–9.

21. Liao WH, Wu HM, Wu HY, et al. Revisiting the relationship of three-dimensional fluid attenuation inversion recovery imaging and hearing outcomes in adults with idiopathic unilateral sudden sensorineural hearing loss. Eur J Radiol 2016;85(12): 2188–94.

22. Gao Z, Chi FL. The clinical value of three-dimensional fluid-attenuated inversion recovery magnetic resonance imaging in patients with idiopathic sudden sensorineural hearing loss: a meta-analysis. Otol Neurotol 2014;35(10):1730–5.

23. Golden E, Krivochenitser R, Mathews N, et al. Contrast-enhanced 3D-FLAIR imaging of the optic nerve and optic nerve head: novel neuroimaging findings of idiopathic intracranial hypertension. AJNR Am J Neuroradiol 2019;40(2):334–9.

24. Fujinaga Y, Kitou Y, Ohya A, et al. Advantages of radial volumetric breath-hold examination (VIBE) with k-space weighted image contrast reconstruction (KWIC) over Cartesian VIBE in liver imaging of volunteers simulating inadequate or no breath-holding ability. Eur Radiol 2016;26(8):2790–7.

25. Wu X, Raz E, Block TK, et al. Contrast-enhanced radial 3D fat-suppressed T1-weighted gradient-recalled echo sequence versus conventional fat-suppressed contrast-enhanced T1-weighted studies of the head and neck. AJR Am J Roentgenol 2014;203(4):883–9.

26. Majigsuren M, Abe T, Kageji T, et al. Comparison of brain tumor contrast-enhancement on T1-CUBE and 3D-SPGR images. Magn Reson Med Sci 2016;15(1): 34–40.

27. Goske MJ, Applegate KE, Boylan J, et al. The Image Gently campaign: working together to change practice. AJR Am J Roentgenol 2008;190(2):273–4.

28. Mayo-Smith WW, Morin RL. Image wisely: the beginning, current status, and future opportunities. J Am Coll Radiol 2017;14(3):442–3.

29. Eley KA, McIntyre AG, Watt-Smith SR, et al. "Black bone" MRI: a partial flip angle technique for radiation reduction in craniofacial imaging. Br J Radiol 2012; 85(1011):272–8.

30. Wiesinger F, Sacolick LI, Menini A, et al. Zero TE MR bone imaging in the head. Magn Reson Med 2016; 75(1):107–14.

31. Wiesinger F, Bylund M, Yang J, et al. Zero TE-based pseudo-CT image conversion in the head and its application in PET/MR attenuation correction and MR-guided radiation therapy planning. Magn Reson Med 2018;80(4):1440–51.

32. Tan AP. MRI protocol for craniosynostosis: replacing ionizing radiation-based CT. AJR Am J Roentgenol 2019;213(6):1374–80.

33. Lu A, Gorny KR, Ho ML. Zero TE MRI for craniofacial bone imaging. AJNR Am J Neuroradiol 2019;40(9):1562–6.

34. Dremmen MHG, Wagner MW, Bosemani T, et al. Does the addition of a "black bone" sequence to a fast multisequence trauma MR protocol allow MRI to replace CT after traumatic brain injury in children? AJNR Am J Neuroradiol 2017;38(11):2187–92.

35. Kralik SF, Supakul N, Wu IC, et al. Black bone MRI with 3D reconstruction for the detection of skull fractures in children with suspected abusive head trauma. Neuroradiology 2019;61(1):81–7.

36. Wendl CM, Eiglsperger J, Dendl LM, et al. Fat suppression in magnetic resonance imaging of the head and neck region: is the two-point DIXON technique superior to spectral fat suppression? Br J Radiol 2018;91(1085):20170078.

37. Delfaut EM, Beltran J, Johnson G, et al. Fat suppression in MR imaging: techniques and pitfalls. Radiographics 1999;19(2):373–82.

38. Krinsky G, Rofsky NM, Weinreb JC. Nonspecificity of short inversion time inversion recovery (STIR) as a technique of fat suppression: pitfalls in image interpretation. AJR Am J Roentgenol 1996;166(3):523–6.

39. Kaldoudi E, Williams SC, Barker GJ, et al. A chemical shift selective inversion recovery sequence for fat-suppressed MRI: theory and experimental validation. Magn Reson Imaging 1993;11(3):341–55.

40. Gaddikeri S, Mossa-Basha M, Andre JB, et al. Optimal fat suppression in head and neck MRI: comparison of multipoint dixon with 2 different fat-suppression techniques, spectral presaturation and inversion recovery, and STIR. AJNR Am J Neuroradiol 2018;39(2):362–8.

41. Reeder SB, Pineda AR, Wen Z, et al. Iterative decomposition of water and fat with echo asymmetry and least-squares estimation (IDEAL): application with fast spin-echo imaging. Magn Reson Med 2005;54(3):636–44.

42. Kralik SF, Haider KM, Lobo RR, et al. Orbital infantile hemangioma and rhabdomyosarcoma in children: differentiation using diffusion-weighted magnetic resonance imaging. J AAPOS 2018;22(1):27–31.

43. Hiwatashi A, Togao O, Yamashita K, et al. Diffusivity of intraorbital lymphoma vs. inflammation: comparison of single shot turbo spin echo and multishot echo planar imaging techniques. Eur Radiol 2018;28(1):325–30.

44. Dremmen MH, Hofman PA, Hof JR, et al. The diagnostic accuracy of non-echo-planar diffusion-weighted imaging in the detection of residual and/or recurrent cholesteatoma of the temporal bone. AJNR Am J Neuroradiol 2012;33(3):439–44.

45. Hatakenaka M, Nakamura K, Yabuuchi H, et al. Pretreatment apparent diffusion coefficient of the primary lesion correlates with local failure in head-and-neck cancer treated with chemoradiotherapy or radiotherapy. Int J Radiat Oncol Biol Phys 2011;81(2):339–45.

46. Connolly M, Srinivasan A. Diffusion-weighted imaging in head and neck cancer: technique, limitations, and applications. Magn Reson Imaging Clin N Am 2018;26(1):121–33.

47. Vandecaveye V, Dirix P, De Keyzer F, et al. Predictive value of diffusion-weighted magnetic resonance imaging during chemoradiotherapy for head and neck squamous cell carcinoma. Eur Radiol 2010;20(7):1703–14.

48. Kim S, Loevner L, Quon H, et al. Diffusion-weighted magnetic resonance imaging for predicting and detecting early response to chemoradiation therapy of squamous cell carcinomas of the head and neck. Clin Cancer Res 2009;15(3):986–94.

49. Bammer R. Basic principles of diffusion-weighted imaging. Eur J Radiol 2003;45(3):169–84.

50. Bae YJ, Choi BS, Jeong HK, et al. Diffusion-weighted imaging of the head and neck: influence of fat-suppression technique and multishot 2D navigated interleaved acquisitions. AJNR Am J Neuroradiol 2018;39(1):145–50.

51. Wang M, Liu H, Wei X, et al. Application of reduced-FOV diffusion-weighted imaging in evaluation of normal pituitary glands and pituitary macroadenomas. AJNR Am J Neuroradiol 2018;39(8):1499–504.

52. Huins CT, Singh A, Lingam RK, et al. Detecting cholesteatoma with non-echo planar (HASTE) diffusion-weighted magnetic resonance imaging. Otolaryngol Head Neck Surg 2010;143(1):141–6.

53. Verhappen MH, Pouwels PJ, Ljumanovic R, et al. Diffusion-weighted MR imaging in head and neck cancer: comparison between half-fourier acquired single-shot turbo spin-echo and EPI techniques. AJNR Am J Neuroradiol 2012;33(7):1239–46.

54. Pipe JG, Farthing VG, Forbes KP. Multishot diffusion-weighted FSE using PROPELLER MRI. Magn Reson Med 2002;47(1):42–52.

55. Mas-Estelles F, Mateos-Fernandez M, Carrascosa-Bisquert B, et al. Contemporary non-echo-planar diffusion-weighted imaging of middle ear cholesteatomas. Radiographics 2012;32(4):1197–213.

56. Iima M, Le Bihan D. Clinical intravoxel incoherent motion and diffusion MR imaging: past, present, and future. Radiology 2016;278(1):13–32.

57. Liang L, Luo X, Lian Z, et al. Lymph node metastasis in head and neck squamous carcinoma: efficacy of

intravoxel incoherent motion magnetic resonance imaging for the differential diagnosis. Eur J Radiol 2017;90:159–65.

58. Ramey NA, Lucarelli MJ, Gentry LR, et al. Clinical usefulness of orbital and facial time-resolved imaging of contrast kinetics (TRICKS) magnetic resonance angiography. Ophthalmic Plast Reconstr Surg 2012;28(5):361–8.

59. Neves F, Huwart L, Jourdan G, et al. Head and neck paragangliomas: value of contrast-enhanced 3D MR angiography. AJNR Am J Neuroradiol 2008;29(5): 883–9.

60. Schicchi N, Tagliati C, Agliata G, et al. MRI evaluation of peripheral vascular anomalies using time-resolved imaging of contrast kinetics (TRICKS) sequence. Radiol Med 2018;123(8):563–71.

61. Razek AA, Gaballa G, Megahed AS, et al. Time resolved imaging of contrast kinetics (TRICKS) MR angiography of arteriovenous malformations of head and neck. Eur J Radiol 2013;82(11):1885–91.

62. Martens RM, Noij DP, Ali M, et al. Functional imaging early during (chemo)radiotherapy for response prediction in head and neck squamous cell carcinoma; a systematic review. Oral Oncol 2019;88:75–83.

63. Korosec FR, Frayne R, Grist TM, et al. Time-resolved contrast-enhanced 3D MR angiography. Magn Reson Med 1996;36(3):345–51.

64. Higgins LJ, Koshy J, Mitchell SE, et al. Time-resolved contrast-enhanced MRA (TWIST) with gadofosveset trisodium in the classification of soft-tissue vascular anomalies in the head and neck in children following updated 2014 ISSVA classification: first report on systematic evaluation of MRI and TWIST in a cohort of 47 children. Clin Radiol 2016;71(1):32–9.

65. Noworolski SM, Fischbein NJ, Kaplan MJ, et al. Challenges in dynamic contrast-enhanced MRI imaging of cervical lymph nodes to detect metastatic disease. J Magn Reson Imaging 2003;17(4):455–62.

66. Bernstein JM, Homer JJ, West CM. Dynamic contrast-enhanced magnetic resonance imaging biomarkers in head and neck cancer: potential to guide treatment? A systematic review. Oral Oncol 2014;50(10):963–70.

67. Kabadi SJ, Fatterpekar GM, Anzai Y, et al. Dynamic contrast-enhanced MR imaging in head and neck cancer. Magn Reson Imaging Clin N Am 2018; 26(1):135–49.

68. Shukla-Dave A, Obuchowski NA, Chenevert TL, et al. Quantitative imaging biomarkers alliance (QIBA) recommendations for improved precision of DWI and DCE-MRI derived biomarkers in multicenter oncology trials. J Magn Reson Imaging 2019;49(7):e101–21.

69. Davis AJ, Rehmani R, Srinivasan A, et al. Perfusion and permeability imaging for head and neck cancer: theory, acquisition, postprocessing, and relevance to clinical imaging. Magn Reson Imaging Clin N Am 2018;26(1):19–35.

70. Saranathan M, Rettmann DW, Hargreaves BA, et al. DIfferential subsampling with Cartesian Ordering (DISCO): a high spatio-temporal resolution Dixon imaging sequence for multiphasic contrast enhanced abdominal imaging. J Magn Reson Imaging 2012; 35(6):1484–92.

71. Feng L, Grimm R, Block KT, et al. Golden-angle radial sparse parallel MRI: combination of compressed sensing, parallel imaging, and golden-angle radial sampling for fast and flexible dynamic volumetric MRI. Magn Reson Med 2014;72(3): 707–17.

72. Deibler AR, Pollock JM, Kraft RA, et al. Arterial spin-labeling in routine clinical practice, part 1: technique and artifacts. AJNR Am J Neuroradiol 2008;29(7): 1228–34.

73. Geerts B, Leclercq D, Tezenas du Montcel S, et al. Characterization of skull base lesions using pseudo-continuous arterial spin labeling. Clin Neuroradiol 2019;29(1):75–86.

74. Yamamoto T, Kimura H, Hayashi K, et al. Pseudo-continuous arterial spin labeling MR images in Warthin tumors and pleomorphic adenomas of the parotid gland: qualitative and quantitative analyses and their correlation with histopathologic and DWI and dynamic contrast enhanced MRI findings. Neuroradiology 2018;60(8):803–12.

75. Fujima N, Kudo K, Yoshida D, et al. Arterial spin labeling to determine tumor viability in head and neck cancer before and after treatment. J Magn Reson Imaging 2014;40(4):920–8.

76. Fujima N, Yoshida D, Sakashita T, et al. Usefulness of pseudocontinuous arterial spin-labeling for the assessment of patients with head and neck squamous cell carcinoma by measuring tumor blood flow in the pretreatment and early treatment period. AJNR Am J Neuroradiol 2016;37(2):342–8.

77. Yanasak NE, Kelly MJ. MR imaging artifacts and parallel imaging techniques with calibration scanning: a new twist on old problems. Radiographics 2014; 34(2):532–48.

78. Kojima T, Yabuuchi H, Narita H, et al. Efficacy of the radial acquisition regime (RADAR) for acquiring head and neck MR images. Br J Radiol 2016; 89(1067):20160007.

79. Lustig M, Donoho D, Pauly JM. Sparse MRI: the application of compressed sensing for rapid MR imaging. Magn Reson Med 2007;58(6):1182–95.

80. Lu SS, Qi M, Zhang X, et al. Clinical evaluation of highly accelerated compressed sensing time-of-flight MR angiography for intracranial arterial stenosis. AJNR Am J Neuroradiol 2018;39(10):1833–8.

81. Yuhasz M, Hoch MJ, Hagiwara M, et al. Accelerated internal auditory canal screening magnetic resonance imaging protocol with compressed sensing

3-dimensional T2-weighted sequence. Invest Radiol 2018;53(12):742–7.

82. Delattre BMA, Boudabbous S, Hansen C, et al. Compressed sensing MRI of different organs: ready for clinical daily practice? Eur Radiol 2020;30(1): 308–19.

83. Rossi Espagnet MC, Bangiyev L, Haber M, et al. High-resolution DCE-MRI of the pituitary gland using radial k-space acquisition with compressed sensing reconstruction. AJNR Am J Neuroradiol 2015;36(8): 1444–9.

84. Mogen JL, Block KT, Bansal NK, et al. Dynamic contrast-enhanced MRI to differentiate parotid neoplasms using golden-angle radial sparse parallel imaging. AJNR Am J Neuroradiol 2019;40(6):1029–36.

85. Bashir U, Mallia A, Stirling J, et al. PET/MRI in oncological imaging: state of the art. Diagnostics (Basel) 2015;5(3):333–57.

86. Liu F, Jang H, Kijowski R, et al. Deep learning MR imaging-based attenuation correction for PET/MR imaging. Radiology 2018;286(2):676–84.

87. Martin O, Schaarschmidt BM, Kirchner J, et al. PET/MRI versus PET/CT in whole-body staging: results from a unicenter observational study in 1003 subsequent examinations. J Nucl Med 2019. https://doi.org/10.2967/jnumed.119.233940.

88. Galgano SJ, Marshall RV, Middlebrooks EH, et al. PET/MR imaging in head and neck cancer: current applications and future directions. Magn Reson Imaging Clin N Am 2018;26(1):167–78.

89. Schwartz DL, Rajendran J, Yueh B, et al. FDG-PET prediction of head and neck squamous cell cancer outcomes. Arch Otolaryngol Head Neck Surg 2004;130(12):1361–7.

90. Chen SW, Hsieh TC, Yen KY, et al. Interim FDG PET/CT for predicting the outcome in patients with head and neck cancer. Laryngoscope 2014;124(12): 2732–8.

91. Lin P, Min M, Lee M, et al. Nodal parameters of FDG PET/CT performed during radiotherapy for locally advanced mucosal primary head and neck squamous cell carcinoma can predict treatment outcomes: SUVmean and response rate are useful imaging biomarkers. Eur J Nucl Med Mol Imaging 2017;44(5):801–11.

92. Min M, Lin P, Lee MT, et al. Prognostic role of metabolic parameters of (18)F-FDG PET-CT scan performed during radiation therapy in locally advanced head and neck squamous cell carcinoma. Eur J Nucl Med Mol Imaging 2015;42(13): 1984–94.

93. Becker M, Varoquaux AD, Combescure C, et al. Local recurrence of squamous cell carcinoma of the head and neck after radio(chemo)therapy: diagnostic performance of FDG-PET/MRI with diffusion-weighted sequences. Eur Radiol 2018;28(2): 651–63.

94. Gallagher TA, Nemeth AJ, Hacein-Bey L. An introduction to the Fourier transform: relationship to MRI. AJR Am J Roentgenol 2008;190(5):1396–405.

95. Chong JJR. Deep-learning super-resolution MRI: getting something from nothing. J Magn Reson Imaging 2020;51(4):1140–1.

96. Hyun CM, Kim HP, Lee SM, et al. Deep learning for undersampled MRI reconstruction. Phys Med Biol 2018;63(13):135007.

97. Lundervold AS, Lundervold A. An overview of deep learning in medical imaging focusing on MRI. Z Med Phys 2019;29(2):102–27.

98. Mazurowski MA, Buda M, Saha A, et al. Deep learning in radiology: an overview of the concepts and a survey of the state of the art with focus on MRI. J Magn Reson Imaging 2019;49(4):939–54.

99. Zhu B, Liu JZ, Cauley SF, et al. Image reconstruction by domain-transform manifold learning. Nature 2018;555(7697):487–92.

Dual Energy Computed Tomography in Head and Neck Imaging: Pushing the Envelope

Thiparom Sananmuang, MD[a,b], Mohit Agarwal, MD[c], Farhad Maleki, PhD[a],
Nikesh Muthukrishnan, MEng[a], Juan Camilo Marquez, MD[a,d],
Jeffrey Chankowsky, MD[d], Reza Forghani, MD, PhD[a,d,e,f,g],*

KEYWORDS

- Dual energy CT • Spectral CT • Head and neck squamous cell carcinoma
- Thyroid cartilage invasion • Radiomics • Texture analysis • Machine learning
- Deep neural networks

KEY POINTS

- Different dual energy computed tomography (DECT) reconstructions can be used to improve diagnostic evaluation of head and neck disorders, especially cancer, compared with conventional single energy computed tomography (CT) scans.
- Different energy DECT virtual monochromatic images and iodine maps can improve tumor visualization, boundary delineation, and accuracy for evaluation of thyroid cartilage invasion.
- Other potential DECT applications include dental artifact reduction, evaluation of lymphadenopathy, and the use of virtual unenhanced images for evaluation of sialolithiasis.
- A multiparametric strategy using a combination of various reconstructed image sets seems to be the optimal DECT approach for head and neck cancer evaluation in the current clinical setting.
- Early evidence suggests that the large amount of quantitative information on DECT scans may be advantageous compared with single energy CT for applications of radiomics and machine learning using quantitative image-based features as biomarkers for tumor characterization and predictive modeling.

Dual energy computed tomography (DECT) is an advanced computed tomography (CT) platform in which attenuation data are acquired at 2 different peak energies instead of 1 peak energy. The acquisition and merging of attenuation data at 2 different energy spectra enables the generation of various image reconstructions and quantitative analysis not possible with standard, single energy CT (SECT) systems. Although interest in DECT dates back to the 1970s, during the early days

[a] Augmented Intelligence & Precision Health Laboratory, Department of Radiology, Research Institute of the McGill University Health Centre, 1001 Decarie Boulevard, Montreal, Quebec H4A 3J1, Canada; [b] Department of Diagnostic and Therapeutic Radiology and Research, Faculty of Medicine, Ramathibodi Hospital, 270 Thanon Rama VI, Thung Phaya Thai, Ratchathewi, Bangkok 10400, Thailand; [c] Department of Radiology, Section of Neuroradiology, Froedtert and Medical College of Wisconsin, Milwaukee, 9200 W Wisconsin Avenue, WI 53226, USA; [d] Department of Radiology, McGill University, 1650 Cedar Avenue, Montreal, Quebec H3G 1A4, Canada; [e] Segal Cancer Centre, Lady Davis Institute for Medical Research, Jewish General Hospital, 3755 Cote Suite-Catherine Road, Montreal, Quebec H3T 1E2, Canada; [f] Gerald Bronfman Department of Oncology, McGill University, Suite 720, 5100 Maisonneuve Boulevard West, Montreal, Quebec H4A3T2, Canada; [g] Department of Otolaryngology, Head and Neck Surgery, Royal Victoria Hospital, McGill University Health Centre, 1001 boul. Decarie Boulevard, Montreal, Quebec H3A 3J1, Canada
* Corresponding author. Department of Radiology, McGill University, 1001 Decarie Boulevard, Montreal, Quebec H3A 3J1, Canada.
E-mail address: reza.forghani@mcgill.ca

Neuroimag Clin N Am 30 (2020) 311–323
https://doi.org/10.1016/j.nic.2020.04.003
1052-5149/20/© 2020 Elsevier Inc. All rights reserved.

following invention of CT, the necessary technological and computational advances for successful clinical implementation of this technology were made many years later, with the introduction of the first clinical DECT scanner in 2006.[1–3] Since its introduction into the clinical arena, numerous DECT applications have emerged in various organ systems. This article reviews the current and emerging applications of DECT for head and neck imaging. The article begins with a brief overview of DECT, followed by various applications of DECT in the head and neck representing largely but not exclusively applications tailored for head and neck oncology. The article concludes by discussing other and emerging applications, and the next steps in the evolution of this technology, including combined applications of radiomics and machine learning for leveraging the large amount of quantitative spectral data available in DECT scans for building clinical prediction models.

DUAL ENERGY COMPUTED TOMOGRAPHY PRINCIPLES, RECONSTRUCTIONS, AND MATERIAL CHARACTERIZATION
Overview

To understand the different applications of DECT, basic familiarity with the underlying principles, common types of DECT reconstructions, and quantitative analytical capabilities of the technology are required. For DECT scanning, attenuation data are acquired at 2 peak energies and combined to generate images for diagnostic interpretation, in contradistinction with SECT, where attenuation data are acquired at 1 peak energy. For optimal DECT scanning, the attenuation data should be obtained simultaneously or near simultaneously and with as little overlap as possible between the 2 energy spectra. This process is achievable with all of the current clinically available premium DECT platforms, including dual-source DECT, rapid kV switching DECT, and layered or sandwich detector DECT (**Fig. 1**). A summary of different approaches for obtaining DECT scans is provided in **Fig. 1**. A more detailed discussion of different DECT approaches and systems as well as their unique advantages and disadvantages is beyond the scope of this article but can be found in recent reviews.[4–6] Note that, in the literature, the term spectral imaging is sometimes used as a substitute for DECT scanning. This usage is not incorrect because DECT scans use attenuation data from 2 different energy spectra, and premium DECT systems enable generation of reconstructions at different energies or characterization of energy-dependent attenuation of a material or

tissue. However, exclusive claims for being the only spectral system by any particular vendor may not be justified because all current clinical DECT scanners, assuming they have not been modified for research purposes, ultimately acquire data at 2 different energy spectra. Therefore, they are all DECT scanners, in contradistinction to other experimental systems that may allow scanning at more than 2 energies.[4,6] Because of their earlier availability, most of the applications discussed in this article are based on investigations using either a rapid kV switching or dual-source DECT scanner. However, these applications are likely at least in part transferable to other DECT systems, although this may require adjustments tailored for the specific platform for optimal use.

Virtual Monochromatic Images and Spectral Hounsfield Unit Attenuation Curves

One type of reconstruction possible with DECT is the virtual monochromatic or monoenergetic image (VMI) (examples shown in **Fig. 2**). These VMIs are created using sophisticated algorithms that combine the attenuation data at the 2 energy spectra and generate images simulating what an image would look like if the scan was acquired at a given or prescribed energy with a monochromatic x-ray beam. The typical range of VMI energy reconstructions that can be generated with current DECT scanners is between 40 kiloelectron volts (keV) and 140 keV or higher depending on the scanner used. The spectral Hounsfield unit attenuation curve (SHUAC) is the quantitative correlate to the VMIs, representing attenuation values at different energies obtained using region of interest (ROI) analysis (**Fig. 3**). The SHUAC is one way to represent the rich quantitative data available in a DECT scan. Unlike SECT, where a ROI would yield 1 average attenuation measurement, ROI analysis of a tissue on a DECT scan can provide a range of measurements at different energies or an attenuation curve[5,7] (see **Fig. 3**). Furthermore, different tissues can have different attenuation curves and this can be exploited in different ways for tissue characterization and diagnostic evaluation[5,7–10] (see **Fig. 3**).

Typically, VMIs reconstructed at 65 or 70 keV are considered similar to a standard 120-kV peak (kVp) SECT scan[9,11–14] and for fast kV switching scanners, VMIs at one of these energies are generated as a default image set for diagnostic interpretation (see **Fig. 2**). As discussed later, many DECT applications are based on the use of VMIs with different energy levels, one example being the use of low-energy VMIs

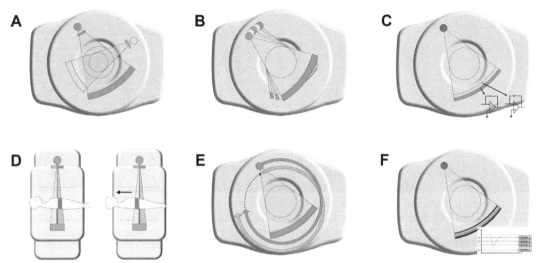

Fig. 1. Different DECT scanners. For optimal DECT scanning, projection data should be obtained simultaneously or near simultaneously at 2 different peak energies, represented by different colors. (*A*) Dual-source DECT (Siemens AG). This system consists of 2 source x-ray tubes with 2 corresponding detectors at a nearly orthogonal angle, enabling the same slice to be imaged simultaneously at high and low energies. (*B*) Single source DECT with rapid kV switching (GE Healthcare). Projection data are collected twice for every projection, 1 at high and 1 at low tube voltage, by very fast switching between low-energy and high-energy spectra combined with fast sampling capabilities of a proprietary, garnet-based scintillator detector with low afterglow for spectral separation at each successive axial or spiral view. (*C*) Dual-layer or sandwich detector DECT (Philips Healthcare). This system consists of a single source and detector, but the detector is composed of 2 scintillation layers. With this system, separation of high-energy and low-energy spectra produced by a single source occurs at the level of the detector. (*D*) TwinBeam DECT (Siemens AG). This system consists of a single source-detector combination in which a split filter at the output of the tube results in separation of the beam into low-energy and high-energy spectra. (*E*) Sequential scanning approach for DECT is one of the earliest and simplest ways to obtain DECT scans. Data at 2 different energies are acquired sequentially at the same positions using different tube voltages. However, there can be significant limitations using this approach because of effects of motion and temporal misregistration that may limit successful use of this technology to certain niche areas. (*F*) A photon-counting scanner, one of the most advanced spectral CT systems currently under development and only available for experimental use at this time. These scanners use photon-counting detectors to resolve the energy of individual photons or photon bins. Theoretically, narrow selectable subranges (or bins) of the spectrum can then be used to classify materials based on their spectral characteristics, enabling multienergy material characterization. (*Adapted from* Forghani R, De Man B, Gupta Rajiv. Dual-Energy Computed Tomography: Physical Principles, Approaches to Scanning, Usage, and Implementation: Part 1. Neuroimag Clin N Am. 2017 Aug;27(3):371-384; with permission.)

to accentuate enhancing tissues (see **Fig. 2**). Iodine, the main constituent of CT contrast agents, has a k-edge of 33.2 keV, which is lower than the 65-keV or 70-keV VMIs typically used as a substitute for a SECT scan. Based on fundamental physical principles, it would be expected that the attenuation of enhancing tissues would increase on low-energy VMIs approaching the k-edge of iodine, as shown qualitatively in **Fig. 2** and quantitatively in **Fig. 3**. This property can be used for oncologic imaging of head and neck squamous cell carcinoma (HNSCC), as discussed later. However, the increased attenuation and soft tissue contrast in this technique typically come at the expense of increased image noise, which can be, at least partly, mitigated either by the use of specialized advanced image reconstruction methods or by optimization of iterative reconstruction settings.[15,16] In addition, with some imaging platforms, such as the layered detector scanner, low-energy VMIs are generated at a low noise level using their proprietary reconstruction algorithms.

Weighted Average Images

Weighted average (WA) images are another type of reconstruction possible with DECT, generated by using a dual-source type of DECT scanner. Typically, a linear blend of 30% of the low-energy and 70% of the high-energy attenuation data is used as a substitute for the standard 120-kVp SECT acquisition and used for routine clinical interpretation.[17–20] Alternative blending combinations as well as different methods of blending (eg, nonlinear) can also be used to accentuate tissue characteristics of interest.[18,21]

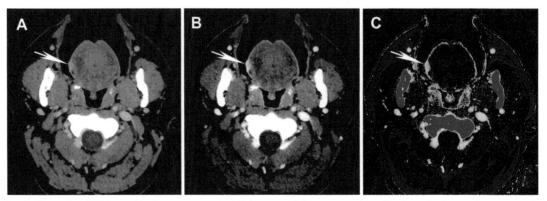

Fig. 2. Example of VMIs and iodine-water material decomposition map and applications for improving tumor visibility: (*A*) 65-keV VMI, typically considered similar to a standard 120-kVp single energy CT image; (*B*) 40-keV VMI; and (*C*) iodine-water map from a patient with a small lateral right oral tongue head and neck squamous cell carcinoma (HNSCC) (*arrows*). Note improved tumor visibility and soft tissue contrast on the low-energy, 40-keV VMI (*B*) compared with the 65-keV VMI (*A*). In this case, the lesion is also well seen and delineated on the iodine map (*C*). The scan was acquired with a fast kVp switching scanner.

Basis Material Decomposition Maps

Basis material decomposition maps are a unique type of image reconstruction possible with DECT and not with SECT.[3,5,6] Depending on the physical properties of the element or material of interest, these images can provide a map of the expected distribution and estimated concentration of a given material. DECT is typically best suited for the decomposition of 2 constituent elements, and this

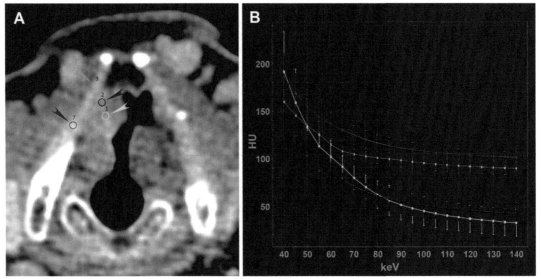

Fig. 3. Example of differences in energy-dependent or spectral characteristics of tissues as shown on SHUACs and its use for discrimination of nonossified thyroid cartilage (NOTC) from tumor. (*A*) Axial 65-keV VMI of a patient with a supraglottic tumor shows ROI analysis of NOTC (*pink/purple*) and tumor (different shades of *blue*). Arrowheads have been placed to help with the visualization of the ROIs. (*B*) SHUACs from the ROI analysis in (*A*). Although the attenuations of NOTC and tumor closely overlap at 65 keV, note how these tissues have different spectral attenuation curves that enable confident discrimination of the 2 types of tissue. More specifically, there is increased separation of the curves in the high-energy range as a result of progressive suppression of iodine within enhancing tumor but relative preservation of the intrinsic high attenuation of NOTC at higher energies. This separation is the basis for the use of high-energy VMIs for distinguishing NOTC from tumor. The scan was acquired with a fast kVp switching scanner. (*Adapted from* Forghani R, Kelly HR, Curtin HD. Applications of Dual-Energy Computed Tomography for the Evaluation of Head and Neck Squamous Cell Carcinoma. Neuroimaging Clin North Am. 2017 Aug;27(3):445-459; with permission.)

type of analysis is performed as a basis pair; for example, iodine-water for generating an iodine map (see **Fig. 2**C) or water-iodine as one of the different possible approaches for creating a virtual noncontrast image from a contrast-enhanced study. Decomposition of more than 2 materials may also be feasible if certain fundamental assumptions are made.[5] Because of its physical properties, iodine is well suited for material decomposition (see **Fig. 2**C). Although material decomposition is a powerful tool, clinicians must be aware of its limitations. First, these maps should not be considered as the physical distribution of a pure element. They are derived from representations based on the physical properties of different materials, which can overlap. For example, calcified tissue or bone has very high signal on iodine maps, as can be readily appreciated in **Fig. 2**C, and should not be misinterpreted as tissue with high iodine content. This pitfall can generally be avoided if the iodine map is interpreted in conjunction with standard reconstructions.

It is not the intent of this article to represent an exhaustive review of the different reconstructions possible with DECT. To stay relevant to the topic, the reconstruction types that are discussed here are the most commonly used for the evaluation of head and neck disorders. DECT applications for head and neck imaging are discussed next.

DUAL ENERGY COMPUTED TOMOGRAPHY APPLICATIONS IN THE HEAD AND NECK
Improving Tumor Visibility and Boundary Discrimination in Head and Neck Squamous Cell Carcinoma

In addition to identifying and characterizing suspected neck abnormalities, one of the essential tasks in the evaluation of HNSCC is to determine the tumor extent. This determination is essential for appropriate tumor staging, and has implications in surgical decision making for extent of tumor resection and in radiation therapy planning to select the appropriate regimen. Multiple retrospective studies using either dual-source DECT or fast kV switching DECT have shown that VMIs reconstructed at energies lower than 65 or 70 keV increase tumor attenuation and soft tissue contrast, consequently improving tumor visualization and soft tissue boundary discrimination[9,11,15,20,22,23] (see **Fig. 2**; **Fig. 4**). Objectively, tumor attenuation is consistently highest at 40 keV, as would be expected based on iodine's energy-dependent attenuation properties and k-edge (see **Fig. 2**). However, in terms of measured contrast to noise ratio and especially subjective preference, there is variation in the preferred low-energy VMIs reported in the literature, ranging between 40 and 60 keV. The discrepancy between the reconstruction with the highest tumor attenuation and subjective preference is likely related to the increased image noise on the 40-keV VMIs.[9,11,15,20,22,23] This discrepancy can likely at least in part be mitigated by advanced methods for generation of low-energy VMIs that have less noise[15] or optimization of adaptive statistical iterative reconstruction settings (Reza Forghani, personal communication, 2020). There is also likely an element of getting accustomed to the noisier 40-keV VMIs through regular use, and it is likely that in studies of subjective preference at least some of the reviewers did not regularly use these reconstructions and therefore may not have been accustomed to these reconstructions. The authors typically use 40-keV VMIs, which are

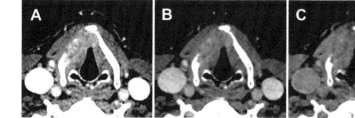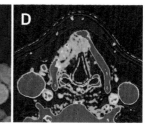

Fig. 4. Examples of VMIs with different energy levels and iodine maps for multiparametric DECT evaluation of thyroid cartilage invasion: (*A*) 40-keV VMI, (*B*) 65-keV VMI, (*C*) 140-keV VMI, and (*D*) iodine-water map reconstructed from DECT of a patient with a right laryngeal HNSCC with through-and-through invasion of the thyroid cartilage. At one extreme, note the increased tumor visibility and soft tissue contrast on the low-energy, 40-keV VMI (*A*) compared with the 65-keV VMI (*B*). At the other extreme, on VMIs reconstructed at a very high energy of 140 keV (*C*), the iodine attenuation has essentially disappeared, approaching what would be expected on an uninfused scan. High-energy VMIs can be especially helpful for discriminating nonossified thyroid cartilage from tumor, as shown in **Fig. 5**. (*D*) Example of an iodine map generated from the same scan, showing the expected distribution and estimated iodine content within enhancing tissues. The scan was acquired with a fast kVp switching scanner. Please refer to article text for additional details.

routinely generated and sent for interpretation in at least 1 of the author's institutions.[24] Although not systematically investigated for this specific purpose, it is the authors' experience that iodine maps can also be helpful for improving tumor visibility and boundary discrimination in some cases (see **Fig. 2**).[25]

Evaluation of Thyroid Cartilage and Thyroid Cartilage Invasion

For the squamous cell carcinoma (SCC) of the larynx and hypopharynx, identification of thyroid cartilage invasion is essential for determining the most appropriate treatment. Functional-preservative partial laryngectomy or chemoradiation have been introduced in the early stage of the disease with limited thyroid cartilage involvement. On the contrary, total laryngectomy is required for selected patients with extensive T3 or large T4a tumors with thyroid cartilage involvement.[26] Evaluation of thyroid cartilage using SECT is challenging because the appearance of the thyroid cartilage on CT varies substantially according to different components of nonossified thyroid cartilage (NOTC), which can have similar attenuation to tumor[8,27–29] (see **Fig. 3**; **Fig. 5**). This variation can become particularly challenging when the tumor is close to or abuts the NOTC. DECT can help make the distinction by taking advantage of differences in energy-dependent attenuation properties of NOTC compared with tumor[8] (see **Figs. 3–5**). Although tumor is better seen on low-energy VMIs because of increasing tumor attenuation, the discrimination from NOTC is best achieved on high-energy VMIs, as shown in a study comparing SHUACs of NOTC and tumor in 30 patients with HNSCC at different primary sites.[8] This difference arises because NOTC does not

enhance and relatively preserves its high attenuation with increasing VMI energy, unlike tumor, which shows suppressed iodine attenuation on increasing energy VMIs moving away from the k-edge of iodine (see **Figs. 3–5**). Based on this study, discrimination and differences in attenuation of NOTC and tumor were most evident at VMI energies of 95 HU or higher.

By using the same principle of vascularized tumor and nonvascularized NOTC, addition of iodine maps to standard SECT equivalent DECT images has also been shown to increase sensitivity for detection of thyroid cartilage invasion without compromising the specificity[30] (see **Figs. 4** and **5**). In a more recent study, it has also been shown that DECT with iodine overlay maps has a higher specificity and acceptable sensitivity in diagnosing laryngeal cartilage invasion compared with magnetic resonance imaging.[31] However, the aim of using iodine maps is to distinguish NOTC from tumor, and ossified thyroid cartilage can have a high signal on iodine maps, which should not be confused with tumor. It must also be ensured that the display settings are correct to avoid false-positive or false-negative designation of iodine content in the area of interest. Interpretation in conjunction with conventional imaging is important and usually enables pitfalls to be recognized.

Dual Energy Computed Tomography for Evaluation and Identification of Tumor Recurrence

On SECT, evaluation of the recurrent tumor on the background of extensive posttreatment change and anatomic distortion can be challenging. As for untreated HNSCC, it has been shown that low-energy VMIs enhance visibility and soft tissue contrast for recurrent tumor.[9,32] In 1 study, it was

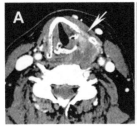 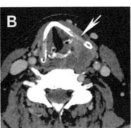 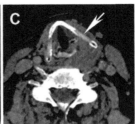 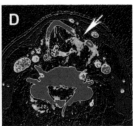

Fig. 5. Examples of VMIs with different energy levels and iodine maps for multiparametric DECT evaluation and distinction of NOTC (*arrow*) from tumor: (*A*) 40-keV VMI, (*B*) 65-keV VMI, (*C*) 140-keV VMI, and (*D*) iodine-water map reconstructed from DECT of a patient with a left hypopharyngeal HNSCC. Note how, at a very high of energy of 140 keV (*C*), the iodine attenuation has essentially disappeared, but the high attenuation of the patch of nearby NOTC is preserved with accentuation of contrast between tumor and NOTC attenuation. This property enables discrimination of NOTC from tumor. (*D*) Example of an iodine map generated from the same scan, showing the absence of significant iodine content in the patch of NOTC. The scan was acquired with a fast kVp switching scanner. Please refer to article text for additional details.

reported that attenuation at 40 KeV and iodine concentration as estimated using iodine maps can distinguish between the posttreatment change and tumor recurrence with 90% specificity and higher accuracy compared with SECT equivalent VMIs at 70 keV.[32] In the authors' experience, another potential benefit of DECT is to use the low-keV VMIs or iodine maps as a screening tool in order to improve the detection of a second primary tumor or for identification of tumor recurrence in patients with treated HNSCC (Fig. 6).

Dual Energy Computed Tomography Applications for the Evaluation of Cervical Lymph Nodes

There are a few studies evaluating the potential advantages of DECT for the characterization of pathologic lymph nodes in the neck. In 1 study using a dual-source type of DECT scanner, the investigators reported that the iodine concentration (mg/mL) and attenuation on iodine overlay (HU) of metastatic HNSCC nodes are significantly lower than in normal or inflammatory lymph nodes.[33] They determined that an optimal iodine concentration threshold value of less than 2.85 mg/mL would enable the diagnosis of nodal metastases with 85% sensitivity and 87.5% specificity.[33]

In a study using a fast kVp switching type of DECT scanner, the investigators evaluated different quantitative parameters for distinguishing nodal metastases from papillary thyroid carcinoma from benign lymph nodes on precontrast, arterial phase, and venous phase acquisitions.[34] Among the various quantitative parameters that were evaluated, venous phase λHU (slope of the SHUAC between 40 keV and 70 keV) and nodal iodine concentration (mg/mL) normalized to that of the left common carotid artery on arterial phase images

increased accuracy for identification of metastatic papillary thyroid carcinoma nodes compared with standard CT parameters.[34] The single best quantitative parameter for detection of metastatic nodes was venous phase λHU, with sensitivity, specificity, accuracy, positive predictive value, and negative predictive value of 62.0%, 91.1%, 80.6%, 79.7%, and 81.0%, respectively. The best combination of quantitative parameters was venous phase λHU and arterial phase normalized iodine concentration, with values of 73.0%, 88.4%, 82.9%, 78.0%, and 85.3%, respectively.[34]

Using similar approaches, other studies have also reported the utility of SHUAC analysis for the characterization of nodal disease. In 1 study comparing metastatic lymph nodes from HNSCC, thyroid carcinoma, salivary carcinoma, and lymphoma, the investigators reported significantly higher iodine concentration (mg/mL) and λHU in thyroid cancer metastases compared with the other nodal pathologies.[35] In addition, the iodine concentration and λHU of the salivary carcinoma group were significantly higher than those of the HNSCC and lymphoma groups.[35] The λHU was calculated as the slope between 40 keV and 90 keV[35] versus 40 and 70 keV in an earlier study.[34] Another study comparing iodine concentration, normalized iodine concentration, and λHU showed statistically significant, higher values in metastatic papillary thyroid cancer lymph nodes compared with normal nodes using a fast kVp switching scanner.[36] The range used to calculate λHU was 40 and 100 keV.

These are some examples of applications of DECT for the characterization of nodal disorder. Although interesting, it would be hard to implement these observations in the clinical setting at this time, and therefore the utility of DECT for nodal characterization in the clinical setting remains to

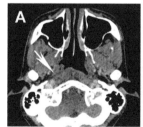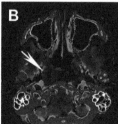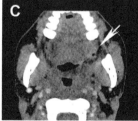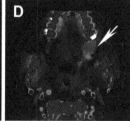

Fig. 6. Example of iodine overlay maps for evaluation of tumor recurrence and screening for second primary tumor. (*A*) Conventional postcontrast axial image at 120 KV and (*B*) iodine overlay map generated from DECT of the patient with treated right-sided nasopharyngeal carcinoma (*arrow, A, B*) showed residual asymmetrical fullness of the right-sided nasopharynx. However, there was also an unexpected second primary tumor (*arrow, C, D*), biopsy proven to be SCC, at the posterior aspect of the left lateral oral tongue that was initially overlooked on conventional postcontrast image at 120 KV (*C*). This tumor was well depicted on the iodine overlay map reconstructed from the DECT (*D*). The scan was acquired using a dual-layer scanner.

be proved. However, if these applications can be automated and incorporated seamlessly into the clinical workflow, there is potential for future impactful incorporation into clinical practice, as discussed at the end of this article.

Other Diagnostic Dual Energy Computed Tomography Applications in the Head and Neck

There are other proposed applications of the DECT for the evaluation of soft tissues of the neck. For example, there is evidence that various quantitative parameters derived from DECT, particularly iodine concentration, may be useful for characterization of the thyroid nodules and distinguishing benign from malignant nodules.[37–40] However, these studies report a variable correlation of the iodine content between benign and malignant nodules, and at this stage their application in the clinical setting requires additional investigations. Other than evaluation of thyroid nodules, a few studies suggest a marginal benefit of DECT for enhancing diagnostic discrimination of parathyroid adenomas from lymph nodes or normal thyroid tissue.[41,42] Virtual unenhanced or noncontrast images derived from a contrast-enhanced neck CT can also be useful for the evaluation of salivary gland stones.[43] Especially considering the variations in CT technique used for the evaluation of sialolithiasis, which could include multiphasic CT performed without and with contrast or just contrast-enhanced neck CT, there is

potential for eliminating the noncontrast acquisition from a multiphasic CT or increasing diagnostic accuracy in practices where only a contrast-enhanced acquisition is obtained for this indication.[43] The neurovascular applications of DECT are beyond the scope of this article and are not discussed.

Metallic Artifact Reduction

For head and neck imaging, dental artifact is one of the most commonly encountered problems for radiologists. Despite the use of several techniques, such as angulation of the CT gantry or an open-mouth view, dental artifact still may obscure part of a lesion and reduce diagnostic quality for tumor evaluation, particularly in the oral cavity and oropharynx. In addition to some degree of inherent artifact reduction in a VMI by virtue of simulating a monochromatic rather than a polychromatic beam acquisition, high-energy VMIs have been shown to reduce the metallic artifact from metallic implants and dental fillings[44–48] (Fig. 7). However, its effectiveness varies depending on the type of dental material and severity of artifact and, as it pertains to dental fillings, typically only modest artifact reduction is seen in areas with significant artifact.[49] Furthermore, this is at the expense of reducing iodine attenuation and therefore tumor visibility and contrast as a major trade-off.[49] In 1 study, VMIs at 95 keV were suggested as a good compromise that may achieve modest metallic artifact reduction (MAR) while preserving sufficient iodine enhancement.[49] Although

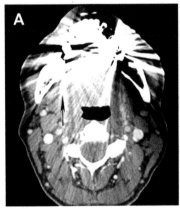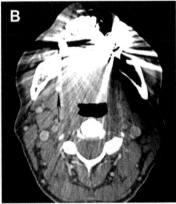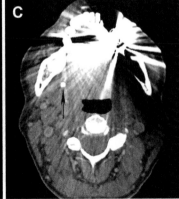

Fig. 7. Dental artifact reduction using high-energy VMIs: (*A*) 65-keV VMI, (*B*) 95-keV VMI, and (*C*) 140-keV VMI reconstructed from the same infused DECT examination show modest artifact reduction on high-energy VMIs at 95 and 140 keV, with the greatest artifact reduction seen on 140-keV VMIs. For example, note how a right submandibular stone (*black arrow*) that cannot be adequately visualized on the 65-keV VMI can be seen on the 95-keV and 140-keV VMIs. The trade-off is suppression of iodine attenuation in enhancing tissues and soft tissue contrast with increasing VMI energies, as can be seen by examination and comparison of normal tissues such as vessels. There is slightly better artifact reduction on the 140-keV compared with the 95-keV VMI; however, the soft tissue contrast is lower. The scan was acquired with a fast kVp switching scanner.

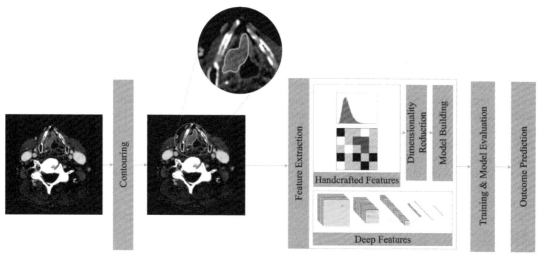

Fig. 8. Overview of the typical radiomic workflow. The major steps in the radiomic workflow consist of lesion identification and localization, segmentation, feature extraction, and prediction model construction. To be adopted in the clinical setting, these have to be seamlessly incorporated into the clinical workflow and automated or semiautomated. Please refer to the article text for additional details.

traditionally MAR has been inconsistent in effectively reducing dental artifact (in contradistinction to some other implants), a combination of high-energy VMIs with MAR reconstruction algorithm has the potential to achieve superior artifact reduction,[44] especially with some of the new DECT platforms incorporating MAR into the reconstruction algorithm (R. Forghani, personal communication). For structures or tissues with intrinsically high attenuation where the suppression of iodine attenuation is not an issue, high-energy VMIs may be more liberally and effectively used; for example, for evaluation of bone or a salivary stone (see **Fig. 7**).

Radiation Therapy Planning

The advantages of DECT discussed earlier are not limited only for diagnostic evaluation. Enhanced tumor visualization and delineation or artifact reduction using DECT has the potential to improve radiation therapy planning and segmentation for treatment of head and neck cancer.[50] Beyond this, DECT has also shown potential for improving dose calculation and planning[51–55] and potentially organ-at-risk segmentation.[56] DECT iodine map–derived quantitative parameters have also shown utility for predicting locoregional recurrence of laryngeal/hypopharyngeal HNSCCs after radiation therapy in a preliminary study.[57] The use of advanced imaging for enhancing personalized therapy in radiation oncology is discussed in greater detail elsewhere (see Monica Shukla and colleagues' article, "Patient-Centric Head and Neck Cancer Radiation Therapy: Role of Advanced Imaging," in this issue).

Emerging Applications of Dual Energy Computed Tomography in Head and Neck Imaging: Radiomics and Machine Learning

During largely qualitative analysis performed in clinical routine practice, there is the potential for underuse of the substantial quantitative information or features available on patients' diagnostic scans. Radiomics was initially defined as the high-throughput extraction of large amounts of features from radiographic images and later extended to encompass the conversion of images to higher-dimensional data and the subsequent mining of these data for improved clinical decision support (**Fig. 8**).[58–60] The features extracted from images can be handcrafted (or hand engineered), meaning that they are derived using predetermined mathematical formulas designed by experts, as done in many of the current radiomics or texture studies. Alternatively, and increasingly, the features extracted from an ROI can represent deep features, meaning that they are learned and derived using deep learning, a type of machine learning. Regardless, such features have shown great potential to be used as quantitative biomarkers for tumor characterization that can be used to predict a variety of clinical or molecular end points of clinical interest.[58,61–66] The use of image extracted features as biomarkers has achieved even greater momentum and potential when combined with machine learning approaches (whether classic machine learning or deep learning) for the development of prediction algorithms. Pertaining to DECT, increasing evidence suggests that the large amount of material-specific quantitative data on these scans can be leveraged using radiomics and machine learning approaches for enhancing prediction model performance for computerized image analysis and/or use of image-based biomarkers.[67–70] Using machine learning, the tissue-specific attenuation curves, such as those shown in **Fig. 3**, can be incorporated into prediction algorithms that use the information for prediction modeling and improve performance compared with images at a single energy.[7,67,69]

In 1 small study using radiomic features from parotid tumors, the use of a similar number of features extracted from VMIs at multiple energies was shown to improve performance compared with features extracted from 65-keV VMIs alone, typically considered similar to a conventional single energy CT scan, with an accuracy of 92% for multienergy analysis compared with 75% for single energy VMI analysis for histopathologic classification of benign parotid tumors.[67] In a more recent study, multienergy radiomics analysis with machine learning was used to extract features from the primary tumor in patients with HNSCC to predict associated nodal metastasis (including micrometastasis), with accuracy of up to 88%, compared with 63% when features extracted at a single VMI energy of 65 keV were used.[69] One exploratory study reported that preradiotherapy analysis of iodine maps of primary gross tumor volume might be useful for prediction of the locoregional recurrence of laryngeal-hypopharyngeal HNSCC.[57] In 1 study using both multienergy and single energy (65 keV) VMI radiomics analysis with machine learning for characterization of pathologic lymph nodes, multienergy analysis did not improve performance.[71] However, the performance at 65-keV VMI was already high, which may have contributed to this. Furthermore, it is expected that the improvements seen will in part depend on the specific disorder of interest. Current investigations of radiomics and/or machine learning for DECT range from basic image processing to advanced tissue characterization and predictive modeling. This issue is an area of active research, and computerized image analysis and machine learning could represent an important area where the potential advantages of DECT compared with conventional SECT are fully realized.

SUMMARY

This article reviews different potential DECT applications in head and neck imaging, concluding with more advanced emerging applications involving radiomics and machine learning. DECT has been shown to have multiple advantages for the evaluation of the head and neck, including for tumor visualization and boundary determination, evaluation of thyroid cartilage invasion, artifact reduction, along with other potential advantages both for the diagnostic evaluation of the head and neck and for radiation therapy planning, which are reviewed here. DECT scans produce rich spectral datasets and new layers of information unavailable in the conventional SECT. However, despite multiple demonstrated advantages of DECT for the evaluation of head and neck (and other organ systems), adoption of the technology in routine clinical practice has been slow, some of which could be related to workflow-related issues that are much better addressed with the newer systems,[24] and some possibly related to marginal perceived benefit. Regardless, it is clear that the extensive quantitative information in DECT scans is underused in the conventional, largely qualitative routine clinical practice. The application of radiomics and artificial intelligence, especially machine learning, has the potential to better leverage this technology's advantages compared with SECT, in addition to the potential for automated analysis, which could make incorporation into clinical practice more seamless and hence increase interest and adoption in busy clinical practices. If the trends in the early studies hold, the combination of emerging computerized image analysis and machine learning applications has the potential to help realize the full potential of DECT to new levels that may then garner much greater and widespread interest and adoption of this technology.

DISCLOSURE

R. Forghani is a clinical research scholar (chercheur-boursier clinicien) supported by the FRQS (Fonds de recherche en santé du Québec). R. Forghani has acted as a consultant and speaker and has a research agreement and research support from GE Healthcare. R. Forghani is also founder and stockholder of 4intelligent Inc.

REFERENCES

1. Flohr TG, McCollough CH, Bruder H, et al. First performance evaluation of a dual-source CT (DSCT) system. Eur Radiol 2006;16:256–68.
2. Johnson TR, Krauss B, Sedlmair M, et al. Material differentiation by dual energy CT: initial experience. Eur Radiol 2007;17:1510–7.
3. Johnson TRC, Kalender WA. Physical background. In: Johnson T, Fink C, Schönberg SO, et al, editors.

Dual energy CT in clinical practice. Berlin: Springer-Verlag Berlin Heidelberg; 2011. p. 3–9.

4. Forghani R, De Man B, Gupta R. Dual-energy computed tomography: physical principles, approaches to scanning, usage, and implementation: part 1. Neuroimaging Clin N Am 2017;27:371–84.

5. Forghani R, De Man B, Gupta R. Dual-energy computed tomography: physical principles, approaches to scanning, usage, and implementation: part 2. Neuroimaging Clin N Am 2017;27:385–400.

6. McCollough CH, Leng S, Yu L, et al. Dual- and multi-energy CT: principles, technical approaches, and clinical applications. Radiology 2015;276:637–53.

7. Forghani R, Srinivasan A, Forghani B. Advanced tissue characterization and texture analysis using dual-energy computed tomography: horizons and emerging applications. Neuroimaging Clin N Am 2017;27:533–46.

8. Forghani R, Levental M, Gupta R, et al. Different spectral hounsfield unit curve and high-energy virtual monochromatic image characteristics of squamous cell carcinoma compared with nonossified thyroid cartilage. AJNR Am J Neuroradiol 2015;36:1194–200.

9. Lam S, Gupta R, Levental M, et al. Optimal virtual monochromatic images for evaluation of normal tissues and head and neck cancer using dual-energy CT. AJNR Am J Neuroradiol 2015;36:1518–24.

10. Srinivasan A, Parker RA, Manjunathan A, et al. Differentiation of benign and malignant neck pathologies: preliminary experience using spectral computed tomography. J Comput Assist Tomogr 2013;37:666–72.

11. Forghani R, Kelly H, Yu E, et al. Low-energy virtual monochromatic dual-energy computed tomography images for the evaluation of head and neck squamous cell carcinoma: a study of tumor visibility compared with single-energy computed tomography and user acceptance. J Comput Assist Tomogr 2017;41:565–71.

12. Matsumoto K, Jinzaki M, Tanami Y, et al. Virtual monochromatic spectral imaging with fast kilovoltage switching: improved image quality as compared with that obtained with conventional 120-kVp CT. Radiology 2011;259:257–62.

13. Patel BN, Thomas JV, Lockhart ME, et al. Single-source dual-energy spectral multidetector CT of pancreatic adenocarcinoma: optimization of energy level viewing significantly increases lesion contrast. Clin Radiol 2013;68:148–54.

14. Pinho DF, Kulkarni NM, Krishnaraj A, et al. Initial experience with single-source dual-energy CT abdominal angiography and comparison with single-energy CT angiography: image quality, enhancement, diagnosis and radiation dose. Eur Radiol 2013;23:351–9.

15. Albrecht MH, Scholtz JE, Kraft J, et al. Assessment of an advanced monoenergetic reconstruction technique in dual-energy computed tomography of head and neck cancer. Eur Radiol 2015;25:2493–501.

16. Forghani R, Kelly HR, Curtin HD. Applications of dual-energy computed tomography for the evaluation of head and neck squamous cell carcinoma. Neuroimaging Clin N Am 2017;27:445–59.

17. Graser A, Johnson TR, Hecht EM, et al. Dual-energy CT in patients suspected of having renal masses: can virtual nonenhanced images replace true nonenhanced images? Radiology 2009;252:433–40.

18. Tawfik AM, Kerl JM, Bauer RW, et al. Dual-energy CT of head and neck cancer: average weighting of low- and high-voltage acquisitions to improve lesion delineation and image quality-initial clinical experience. Invest Radiol 2012;47:306–11.

19. Tawfik AM, Kerl JM, Razek AA, et al. Image quality and radiation dose of dual-energy CT of the head and neck compared with a standard 120-kVp acquisition. AJNR Am J Neuroradiol 2011;32:1994–9.

20. Wichmann JL, Noske EM, Kraft J, et al. Virtual monoenergetic dual-energy computed tomography: optimization of kiloelectron volt settings in head and neck cancer. Invest Radiol 2014;49:735–41.

21. Scholtz JE, Husers K, Kaup M, et al. Non-linear image blending improves visualization of head and neck primary squamous cell carcinoma compared to linear blending in dual-energy CT. Clin Radiol 2015;70:168–75.

22. Kraft M, Ibrahim M, Spector M, et al. Comparison of virtual monochromatic series, iodine overlay maps, and single energy CT equivalent images in head and neck cancer conspicuity. Clin Imaging 2018;48:26–31.

23. May MS, Bruegel J, Brand M, et al. Computed tomography of the head and neck region for tumor staging-comparison of dual-source, dual-energy and low-kilovolt, single-energy acquisitions. Invest Radiol 2017;52:522–8.

24. Perez-Lara A, Levental M, Rosenbloom L, et al. Routine dual-energy computed tomography scanning of the neck in clinical practice: a single-institution experience. Neuroimaging Clin N Am 2017;27:523–31.

25. Perez-Lara A, Forghani R. Dual-energy computed tomography of the neck: a pictorial review of normal anatomy, variants, and pathologic entities using different energy reconstructions and material decomposition maps. Neuroimaging Clin N Am 2017;27:499–522.

26. Forastiere AA, Ismaila N, Lewin JS, et al. Use of larynx-preservation strategies in the treatment of laryngeal cancer: American Society of Clinical

Oncology Clinical Practice Guideline Update. J Clin Oncol 2018;36:1143–69.

27. Becker M, Zbaren P, Delavelle J, et al. Neoplastic invasion of the laryngeal cartilage: reassessment of criteria for diagnosis at CT. Radiology 1997;203: 521–32.

28. Dadfar N, Seyyedi M, Forghani R, et al. Computed tomography appearance of normal nonossified thyroid cartilage: implication for tumor invasion diagnosis. J Comput Assist Tomogr 2015;39:240–3.

29. Hermans R. Staging of laryngeal and hypopharyngeal cancer: value of imaging studies. Eur Radiol 2006;16:2386–400.

30. Kuno H, Onaya H, Iwata R, et al. Evaluation of cartilage invasion by laryngeal and hypopharyngeal squamous cell carcinoma with dual-energy CT. Radiology 2012;265:488–96.

31. Kuno H, Sakamaki K, Fujii S, et al. Comparison of MR imaging and dual-energy CT for the evaluation of cartilage invasion by laryngeal and hypopharyngeal squamous cell carcinoma. AJNR Am J Neuroradiol 2018;39:524–31.

32. Yamauchi H, Buehler M, Goodsitt MM, et al. Dual-energy CT-based differentiation of benign posttreatment changes from primary or recurrent malignancy of the head and neck: comparison of spectral hounsfield units at 40 and 70 keV and iodine concentration. AJR Am J Roentgenol 2016; 206:580–7.

33. Tawfik AM, Razek AA, Kerl JM, et al. Comparison of dual-energy CT-derived iodine content and iodine overlay of normal, inflammatory and metastatic squamous cell carcinoma cervical lymph nodes. Eur Radiol 2014;24:574–80.

34. Liu X, Ouyang D, Li H, et al. Papillary thyroid cancer: dual-energy spectral CT quantitative parameters for preoperative diagnosis of metastasis to the cervical lymph nodes. Radiology 2015;275:167–76.

35. Yang L, Luo D, Li L, et al. Differentiation of malignant cervical lymphadenopathy by dual-energy CT: a preliminary analysis. Sci Rep 2016;6:31020.

36. Zhao Y, Li X, Li L, et al. Preliminary study on the diagnostic value of single-source dual-energy CT in diagnosing cervical lymph node metastasis of thyroid carcinoma. J Thorac Dis 2017;9:4758–66.

37. Gao SY, Zhang XY, Wei W, et al. Identification of benign and malignant thyroid nodules by in vivo iodine concentration measurement using single-source dual energy CT: A retrospective diagnostic accuracy study. Medicine (Baltimore) 2016;95: e4816.

38. Lee DH, Lee YH, Seo HS, et al. Dual-energy CT iodine quantification for characterizing focal thyroid lesions. Head Neck 2019;41:1024–31.

39. Li HW, Wu XW, Liu B, et al. Clinical values of of gemstone spectral CT in diagnosing thyroid disease. J Xray Sci Technol 2015;23:45–56.

40. Li M, Zheng X, Li J, et al. Dual-energy computed tomography imaging of thyroid nodule specimens: comparison with pathologic findings. Invest Radiol 2012;47:58–64.

41. Forghani R, Roskies M, Liu X, et al. Dual-energy CT characteristics of parathyroid adenomas on 25-and 55-second 4D-CT acquisitions: preliminary experience. J Comput Assist Tomogr 2016;40:806–14.

42. Roskies M, Liu X, Hier MP, et al. 3-phase dual-energy CT scan as a feasible salvage imaging modality for the identification of non-localizing parathyroid adenomas: a prospective study. J Otolaryngol Head Neck Surg 2015;44:44.

43. Beland B, Levental M, Srinivasan A, et al. Practice variations in salivary gland imaging and utility of virtual unenhanced dual energy CT images for the detection of major salivary gland stones. Acta Radiol 2018. https://doi.org/10.1177/0284185118817906. 284185118817906.

44. Cha J, Kim HJ, Kim ST, et al. Dual-energy CT with virtual monochromatic images and metal artifact reduction software for reducing metallic dental artifacts. Acta Radiol 2017;58:1312–9.

45. De Crop A, Casselman J, Van Hoof T, et al. Analysis of metal artifact reduction tools for dental hardware in CT scans of the oral cavity: kVp, iterative reconstruction, dual-energy CT, metal artifact reduction software: does it make a difference? Neuroradiology 2015;57:841–9.

46. Grosse Hokamp N, Laukamp KR, Lennartz S, et al. Artifact reduction from dental implants using virtual monoenergetic reconstructions from novel spectral detector CT. Eur J Radiol 2018;104:136–42.

47. Schwahofer A, Bar E, Kuchenbecker S, et al. The application of metal artifact reduction (MAR) in CT scans for radiation oncology by monoenergetic extrapolation with a DECT scanner. Z Med Phys 2015;25:314–25.

48. Tanaka R, Hayashi T, Ike M, et al. Reduction of dark-band-like metal artifacts caused by dental implant bodies using hypothetical monoenergetic imaging after dual-energy computed tomography. Oral Surg Oral Med Oral Pathol Oral Radiol 2013; 115:833–8.

49. Nair JR, DeBlois F, Ong T, et al. Dual-Energy CT: balance between iodine attenuation and artifact reduction for the evaluation of head and neck cancer. J Comput Assist Tomogr 2017. https://doi.org/10. 1097/RCT.0000000000000617.

50. Forghani R. An update on advanced dual-energy CT for head and neck cancer imaging. Expert Rev Anticancer Ther 2019;19:633–44.

51. Almeida IP, Schyns L, Vaniqui A, et al. Monte Carlo proton dose calculations using a radiotherapy specific dual-energy CT scanner for tissue segmentation and range assessment. Phys Med Biol 2018; 63:115008.

52. Bazalova M, Carrier JF, Beaulieu L, et al. Dual-energy CT-based material extraction for tissue segmentation in Monte Carlo dose calculations. Phys Med Biol 2008;53:2439–56.

53. Hunemohr N, Krauss B, Dinkel J, et al. Ion range estimation by using dual energy computed tomography. Z Med Phys 2013;23:300–13.

54. van Elmpt W, Landry G, Das M, et al. Dual energy CT in radiotherapy: current applications and future outlook. Radiother Oncol 2016;119:137–44.

55. Wohlfahrt P, Mohler C, Stutzer K, et al. Dual-energy CT based proton range prediction in head and pelvic tumor patients. Radiother Oncol 2017;125:526–33.

56. Wang T, Ghavidel BB, Beitler JJ, et al. Optimal virtual monoenergetic image in "TwinBeam" dual-energy CT for organs-at-risk delineation based on contrast-noise-ratio in head-and-neck radiotherapy. J Appl Clin Med Phys 2019;20:121–8.

57. Bahig H, Lapointe A, Bedwani S, et al. Dual-energy computed tomography for prediction of loco-regional recurrence after radiotherapy in larynx and hypopharynx squamous cell carcinoma. Eur J Radiol 2019;110:1–6.

58. Gillies RJ, Kinahan PE, Hricak H. Radiomics: images are more than pictures, they are data. Radiology 2016;278:563–77.

59. Kumar V, Gu Y, Basu S, et al. Radiomics: the process and the challenges. Magn Reson Imaging 2012;30:1234–48.

60. Lambin P, Rios-Velazquez E, Leijenaar R, et al. Radiomics: extracting more information from medical images using advanced feature analysis. Eur J Cancer 2012;48:441–6.

61. Aerts HJ, Velazquez ER, Leijenaar RT, et al. Decoding tumour phenotype by noninvasive imaging using a quantitative radiomics approach. Nat Commun 2014;5:4006.

62. Forghani R, Savadjiev P, Chatterjee A, et al. Radiomics and artificial intelligence for biomarker and prediction model development in oncology. Comput Struct Biotechnol J 2019;17:995–1008.

63. Ganeshan B, Panayiotou E, Burnand K, et al. Tumour heterogeneity in non-small cell lung carcinoma assessed by CT texture analysis: a potential marker of survival. Eur Radiol 2012;22:796–802.

64. Lambin P, Leijenaar RTH, Deist TM, et al. Radiomics: the bridge between medical imaging and personalized medicine. Nat Rev Clin Oncol 2017;14:749–62.

65. Lubner MG, Smith AD, Sandrasegaran K, et al. CT texture analysis: definitions, applications, biologic correlates, and challenges. Radiographics 2017;37:1483–503.

66. Parmar C, Leijenaar RT, Grossmann P, et al. Radiomic feature clusters and prognostic signatures specific for Lung and Head & Neck cancer. Sci Rep 2015;5:11044.

67. Al Ajmi E, Forghani B, Reinhold C, et al. Spectral multi-energy CT texture analysis with machine learning for tissue classification: an investigation using classification of benign parotid tumours as a testing paradigm. Eur Radiol 2018;28:2604–11.

68. Foncubierta-Rodriguez A, Jimenez del Toro OA, Platon A, et al. Benefits of texture analysis of dual energy CT for Computer-Aided pulmonary embolism detection. Conf Proc IEEE Eng Med Biol Soc 2013;2013:3973–6.

69. Forghani R, Chatterjee A, Reinhold C, et al. Head and neck squamous cell carcinoma: prediction of cervical lymph node metastasis by dual-energy CT texture analysis with machine learning. Eur Radiol 2019;29:6172–81.

70. Oldan J, He M, Wu T, et al. Pilot study: evaluation of dual-energy computed tomography measurement strategies for positron emission tomography correlation in pancreatic adenocarcinoma. J Digit Imaging 2014;27:824–32.

71. Seidler M, Forghani B, Reinhold C, et al. Dual-Energy CT texture analysis with machine learning for the evaluation and characterization of cervical lymphadenopathy. Comput Struct Biotechnol J 2019;17:1009–15.

PET Imaging of Tumor Hypoxia in Head and Neck Cancer: A Primer for Neuroradiologists

Rihan Khan, MD*, Marc Seltzer, MD

KEYWORDS

• PET • Tumor hypoxia • Head and neck cancer • Imaging

KEY POINTS

- Tumor hypoxia is a known independent prognostic factor for adverse patient outcomes.
- Areas of tumor hypoxia have been found to be more radiation resistant than areas of tumor with normal oxygenation levels.
- Hypoxia imaging may serve to help identify the best initial treatment option and to assess intratreatment monitoring of tumor response in case treatment changes can be made.
- PET imaging is the gold standard method for imaging tumor hypoxia with 18F-fluoromisonidazole the most extensively studied hypoxic imaging tracer.
- Newer tracers that also show promise include 18F-fluoroazomycinarabinoside, 18F-fluoroerythronitroimidazole, 18F-2-nitroimidazol-pentafluoropropyl acetamide, and 18F-flortanidazole.

INTRODUCTION

Tumor hypoxia is a known independent prognostic factor for adverse patient outcomes because areas of tumor hypoxia have been found to be more radiation resistant than areas of tumor with normal oxygenation levels.[1,2] Tumor hypoxia has been shown to be about 75% per patient and 61% per tumor according to PET studies evaluating hypoxic markers.[3,4] Limited oxygen diffusion into the tumor core can cause chronic tumor hypoxia, which is more or less stable, but this can be managed with fractionated radiotherapy, which induces reoxygenation. Oxygen radicals are necessary to cause DNA damage induced by chemotherapy and radiotherapy. The concept of tumor reoxygenation refers to the idea that radiation kills tumor cells that are well oxygenated, thus decreasing the overall local oxygen demand within the entirety of the residual tumor. In theory, the persistent hypoxic tumor cells then have the chance to extract more local oxygen because there is less competition to do so after the previously oxygen-rich tumor cells are killed. Therefore, hypoxic tumor cells may then reoxygenate in time for the next fraction of radiation.[5]

However, acute hypoxia has limited oxygen perfusion as the main cause, which is more unpredictable. Abnormal tumor vasculature often has tortuous vessels, shunting, leaky vessels, and blocked passages that cause a temporary state of hypoxia, which is one reason why biopsies are often not reliable in quantifying tumor hypoxia.[4] The optimum technique to measure tissue oxygen pressures (P_{O_2}) is directly using a polarographic oxygen electrode, but this is an invasive technique and may alter the local tissue oxygen concentration.[1,4] For this reason, noninvasive techniques are desirable to detect tumor hypoxia.

CORRELATION WITH HYPOXIA-SPECIFIC MOLECULAR BIOMARKERS

When evaluating functional imaging biomarkers for treatment response, many studies have compared them with reference standard hypoxia-specific

Department of Radiology, Dartmouth-Hitchcock Medical Center, 1 Medical Center Drive, Lebanon, NH 03756, USA
* Corresponding author.
E-mail address: rihan.khan@hitchcock.org

Neuroimag Clin N Am 30 (2020) 325–339
https://doi.org/10.1016/j.nic.2020.05.003
1052-5149/20/© 2020 Elsevier Inc. All rights reserved.

molecular biomarkers. Specifically with head and neck cancer, the molecular markers hypoxia-inducible factor (HIF-1), carbonic anhydrase IX (CA-IX), and glucose transporter 1 (GLUT-1) are associated with a poor outcome, almost regardless of treatment.[2,4,6]

Regarding imaging biomarkers, many clinicians consider PET to be the gold standard method for hypoxia imaging. 18F-fluoromisonidazole (FMISO) and 18F-fluoroazomycinarabinoside (FAZA) are two of the most commonly used hypoxia-associated tracers, with FMISO-PET regarded as the standard noninvasive modality for hypoxic imaging.[1,7] FMISO-PET was the first in vivo radiotracer, and is the most commonly used radiotracer for in vivo tumor hypoxia imaging. Although popular, FMISO has shown varying results when correlating with tumor markers, uptake, and outcome.[4]

One study of 23 patients with primary oral squamous cell carcinoma showed a significantly higher maximum standardized uptake value (SUVmax) of FMISO in patients positive for HIF-1 than in patients negative for HIF-1, with no significant correlation between 18F-fluorodeoxyglucose (FDG) PET SUVmax and HIF-1. The investigators concluded that FMISO uptake in such patients indicates a hypoxic environment with HIF-1 expression and that both FMISO and HIF-1 are key features of hypoxia.[8] A different study of 24 patients with head and neck cancer examined several factors, including FMISO maximum tumor/venous blood ratios (T/Bmax) and hypoxic tumor volumes compared with HIF-1 and p53 on immunohistochemistry, with hypoxia defined as a T/B ratio of greater than or equal to 1.2. The investigators found a weak correlation between FMISO hypoxic volume and both HIF-1 and p53.[9] A small prospective study of 16 patients with locally advanced head and neck cancer sought to examine the correlation between biological imaging (FMISO-PET) and biological markers (CA-IX, CD44 [cluster of differentiation 44], and Ku80) in a group of patients in whom this correlation had already been shown. However, they found no correlation between the biological markers or with the FMISO-PET imaging variables. However, CA-IX did show a significant association with improved overall survival. They also found a significant negative correlation between CD44 and human papilloma virus (HPV) status.[6]

TRACER REPRODUCIBILITY AND VASCULAR CLEARANCE CONSIDERATIONS

Reproducibility of tracer activity is of prime importance in order to use it in the clinical realm to characterize and follow tumor uptake. Because tumors are known to have areas of both acute and chronic hypoxia, with the acutely hypoxic areas more prone to rapid shifting in oxygen content, a prospective study was performed to determine the reproducibility of FMISO detection in 11 patients with head and neck cancer using serial FMISO-PET imaging 48 hours apart. Each cohort was scanned at 4 hours after tracer injection to standardize tracer uptake and SUVmax, tumor/blood and tumor/muscle (T/M) ratios, tumor volumes, and hypoxic location were examined. FMISO values and tumor volumes were highly reproducible,[10] which was consistent with the results shown in simulation studies.[11]

The biological half-life of FMISO, about 50 minutes, is a notable limitation of the tracer. This half-life is related to FMISO's high lipophilicity, which results in slow plasma clearance. Because of this, delayed imaging at several hours after tracer injection, at least 2 hours and ideally about 4 hours, is necessary for clearance of tracer outside of hypoxic tumor and hypoxic tissue uptake, to obtain better contrast between hypoxic and well-oxygenated tissue.[5,12] Despite some studies having shown a 4-hour postinjection study to be optimal, many of the studies with repeat measurements for patients undergoing radiotherapy have been performed at 2 hours. In order for FMISO imaging to have broad clinical implementation, a standard protocol is necessary.[5] Recently, a study of 18 patients with head and neck squamous cell carcinoma were examined regarding the timing of FMISO tracer uptake measurement to optimize hypoxic tumor volumes. The investigators found that contrast resolution increases with time with a reduction in background activity and increased hypoxic tumor volume. Mean SUV of background activity showed a statistically significant difference between both the 1-hour and 3-hour scans and the 1-hour and 5 hour scans. In addition, mean hypoxic tumor volume progressively increased between the 1-hour, 3-hour, and 5-hour scans, and significantly so between the 1-hour and 3-hour scans and the 1-hour and 5-hour scans.[13]

POTENTIAL CLINICAL APPLICATIONS

Despite mixed results correlating hypoxia-specific molecular markers and FMISO, FMISO has been studied with promising results in a variety of clinical applications. In addition to assessing posttreatment response, hypoxia imaging may serve to help identify the best initial treatment option and to assess intratreatment monitoring of tumor response in case treatment changes can be made.[4]

Determining the Best Initial Treatment Option

In patients with head and neck cancer, increased tumor uptake of FMISO is associated with recurrence, is a poor prognostic factor for overall survival, and multiple studies have shown the value of FMISO-PET for clinical management[5,12] (Fig. 1). A prospective study of 22 patients with oral squamous cell carcinoma undergoing

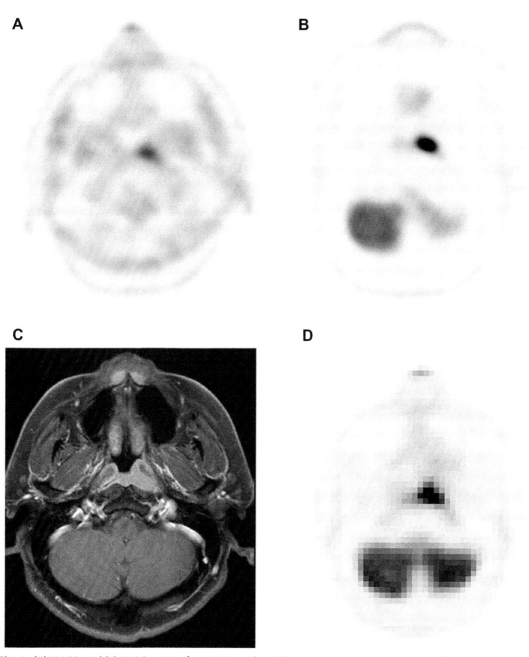

Fig. 1. (A) FMISO and (B) FDG images of a patient with a left nasopharyngeal cancer showed the focal uptakes of both tracers in the tumor. (C) A corresponding slice of a gadolinium-enhanced magnetic resonance (MR) image. (D) Despite a small tumor, positive FMISO uptake and FDG uptake was noted indicating a hypoxic and metabolically active tumor. Six months after the chemoradiotherapy, strong FDG uptake in the area of pretreatment FMISO uptake is noted, indicating tumor recurrence in the hypoxic areas. (*From* Tamaki N, Hirata K. Tumor hypoxia: a new PET imaging biomarker in clinical oncology. Int J Clin Oncol. 2016;21(4):619–625; with permission. (Figure 2 in original).)

preoperative chemotherapy was performed, using both FMISO and FDG-PET. Operative histology was used to measure response. Patients with a negative FMISO-PET scan had a significantly better outcome than those with a positive scan. In addition, no significant correlation was found between the FDG-PET scan and the response to chemotherapy. Thus, overall the study found that FMISO-PET is advantageous in determining a response to chemotherapy in this patient group compared with FDG-PET.[12,14] A different study concluded that tumor hypoxic volume may predict outcomes in patients with oral squamous cell carcinoma. Twenty-three such patients had both FDG-PET/computed tomography (CT) and FMISO-PET/CT before radical surgery and were followed for more than 5 years. Hypoxic tumor volume correlated significantly with both disease-free survival (DFS) and locoregional recurrence, whereas total lesional glycolysis was significantly associated with DFS[15] (**Fig. 2**).

Given that hypoxic tumor volumes are associated with poor outcomes and nonhypoxic tumor with better outcomes, treatment strategies may be tailored to the type of tumor present. This ability has led to studies of radiotherapy dose escalation for hypoxic tumors and studies of dose reduction for nonhypoxic tumors.[12]

Dose De-escalation

Because radiation therapy–related toxicities can be significant, a substudy of 33 patients with HPV-positive oropharyngeal cancer from a larger prospective study assessed pretreatment tumor hypoxia to see whether radiation dose de-escalation could be performed safely. Ten of the patients met criteria for dose reduction from 70 Gy to 60 Gy to the lymph nodes (primary tumor dose remained at 70 Gy), with pretreatment dynamic and static FMISO-PET–positive tumor hypoxia that resolved on a 1-week follow-up FMISO-PET scan after chemoradiation (**Fig. 3**). The 2-

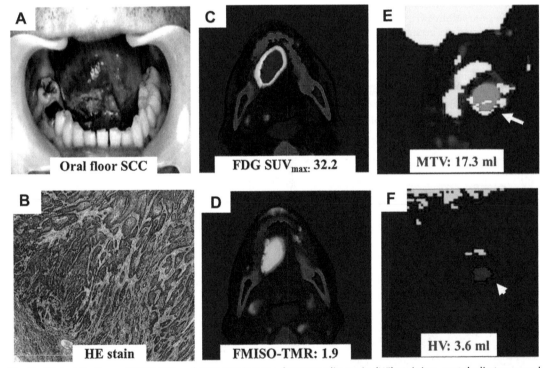

Fig. 2. Clinical findings, FMISO-PET and FDG-PET images, hematoxylin-eosin (HE) staining, metabolic tumor volume (MTV), and hypoxic volume (HV). (*A*) An oral squamous cell carcinoma (SCC) in the right oral floor region. (*B*) Tissue sample stained with HE, showing a keratinized, spindle-shaped nest of invasive cancer cells. (*C*) FDG-PET, showing FDG uptake by the primary tumor in the right oral floor (SUVmax, 32.2). (*D*) FMISO-PET, showing FMISO uptake by the primary tumor (T/M ratio [TMR], 1.9). (*E*) Sagittal image showing the MTV of the primary lesion as a red area 17.3 mL in volume (*arrow*). (*F*) Sagittal image showing the HV of the tumor as a red area 3.6 mL in volume (*arrowhead*). (*From* Sato J, et al. Hypoxic volume evaluated by 18F-fluoromisonidazole positron emission tomography (FMISO-PET) may be a prognostic factor in patients with oral squamous cell carcinoma: preliminary analyses. Int. J. Oral Maxillofac. Surg. 2018;47(5):553–560; with permission. (Figure 1 in original).)

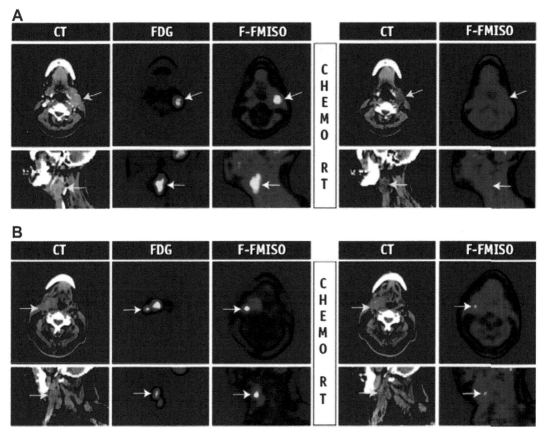

Fig. 3. (*A*) Patient with hypoxia on pretreatment FMISO-PET and with resolution on FMISO$_{1week}$-PET. (*B*) A patient with hypoxia on pretreatment FMISO-PET and persistent hypoxia on FMISO$_{1week}$-PET. RT, radiation therapy. (*From* Lee N, et al. Strategy of Using Intratreatment Hypoxia Imaging to Selectively and Safely Guide Radiation Dose De-escalation Concurrent With Chemotherapy for Locoregionally Advanced Human Papilloma Virus Related Oropharyngeal Carcinoma. Int J Radiation Oncol Biol Phys. 2016;96(1):9-17; with permission. (Figure 2 in original).)

year locoregional control rate in these 10 patients was 100%, suggesting that functional intratreatment FMISO tumor hypoxia imaging may be a safe option as a radiation dose de-escalation strategy.[16]

Dose Escalation

Laboratory studies have shown that up to 3 times the radiation dose is needed to cause cytotoxic effects in hypoxic tumor cells compared with nonhypoxic tumor cells. However, clinical radiation doses are limited because of side effects in normal tissues. Considering this, modestly higher dose escalation to areas of chronically hypoxic tumor have shown improved tumor control.[17]

Ten patients with head and neck squamous cell carcinoma were randomly selected out of a 102-patient cohort, for a subanalysis for dose escalation. FMISO was used to determine hypoxic tumor volumes for boost planning and intensity modulated radiation therapy was used for dose escalation while keeping the radiation dose under the clinically acceptable limits for critical structures. This combination allowed an increased tumor control probability of 17% without an increased risk of expected complications. This hypoxic volume–based approach has been researched in several other studies of head and neck cancer and not only shown to be feasible but also considered superior to uniform radiation dose prescription.[18–21]

A prospective, phase 2, randomized clinical trial was designed to evaluate hypoxia-guided dose escalation based on dynamic FMISO imaging in 80 patients with locally advanced head and neck squamous cell carcinoma (oropharynx or hypopharynx). The dynamic scan entailed 40 minutes of imaging, and static scans were performed at 2 and 4 hours after injection for 15 minutes each. Patients with tumor hypoxia were randomly assigned to standard chemoradiation therapy or dose

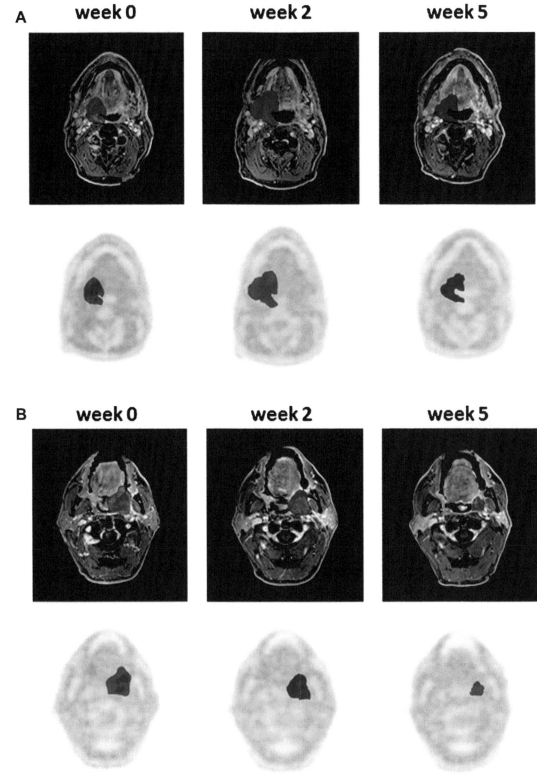

Fig. 4. Representative images showing the differential dynamics of tumor and hypoxic subvolumes during the course of chemoradiation. (*A*) Time course of tumor volumes (*red contours*) and hypoxic tumor subvolumes

escalation to the hypoxic tumor volume, whereas those patients with nonhypoxic tumors received standard chemoradiation therapy. The 2-year local-regional control rate in the hypoxic tumor groups was 44.4% for those receiving standard therapy and 70% for those receiving dose escalation, whereas the nonhypoxic tumor group that underwent standard therapy had a 100% 2-year local-regional control rate. In addition, acute and late toxicity and treatment compliance did not differ significantly between the standard-dose and dose-escalation groups. Thus the investigators concluded that dose escalation may be feasible without increased toxicity.[22]

Intratreatment Monitoring

Studies have suggested that residual hypoxia as indicated by FMISO uptake during chemoradiation therapy may portend a worse prognosis. A prospective study of 49 patients with locally advanced head and neck squamous cell carcinoma who were being treated with chemoradiation had both FDG-PET and FMISO-PET scans at 0, 2, and 5 weeks during treatment and there was a significant correlation between high HIF1-alpha levels and increased tumor hypoxia at the 2-week scan, examining the FMISO tumor/background ratios.[23] (Fig. 4) A different prospective trial reported final results after examining tumor hypoxia in patients with head and neck cancer undergoing primary chemoradiation, examining both FDG-PET and FMISO-PET imaging. The investigators concluded that residual tumor hypoxia in this patient population is a major reason for therapy resistance and that hypoxia noted by FMISO-PET after 2 weeks of chemoradiation therapy may be a biomarker to identify those patients at high risk for locoregional recurrence.[24] A cohort of 25 patients with head and neck cancer with stage 3 or 4 disease prospectively underwent baseline and 3 subsequent intratreatment FMISO-PET scans during chemoradiotherapy (end of weeks 1 and 2, and during week 5). For each scan, imaging was performed at 2 and 4 hours after injection and multiple parameters were assessed, including tumor/background ratio, with background activity measured in the deep neck musculature. An FDG-PET scan was also obtained before chemoradiation. FMISO parameters had a strong association with local progression-free survival (LPFS), strongest at weeks 1 and 2, whereas FDG-PET volumes showed no significant association with LPFS. The investigators concluded that FMISO imaging at weeks 1 and 2 of treatment may be useful to select patients for modification of treatment.[25]

One recent review article from 2018 noted that 12 studies using FMISO-PET, 2 with FAZA, and 1 with HX4 (18F-flortanidazole) examined hypoxia during radiotherapy for head and neck cancer, and all showed decreased tumor hypoxia during therapy. Considering all 15 studies, for those patients with baseline hypoxia, the hypoxia resolved in 33% to 100% of patients between weeks 2 and 5, and, if hypoxia was still present, the volume of hypoxic tissue decreased from a maximum at baseline of 54% to a maximum of 20% at 2 weeks after initiation of treatment. Thus, intratreatment monitoring of tumor hypoxia can reveal which tumors undergo reoxygenation and may have a better response to chemoradiation, and it can also show which tumors will not reoxygenate, indicating a worse prognosis for those patients.[5]

ADDITIONAL HYPOXIC IMAGING TRACERS
18F-fluoroazomycinarabinoside Imaging

Because FMISO tracer uptake into hypoxic tissues and its clearance from the normoxic tissues are both slow, this requires a delay before imaging of up to 4 hours. This limitation is one of the reasons why second-generation nitroimidazole tracers were developed, such as FAZA, with better kinetics.[26] Advantages of FAZA include easy tracer production with high specific activity, postinjection chemical stability, specific metabolism in hypoxic cells, and higher tumor/background ratios because of unbound tracer being rapidly cleared from normoxic tissues,[27] owing to a lower lipophilicity compared with FMISO.[5] FAZA is the second most popular PET imaging tracer for hypoxia after FMISO.[4]

In a prospective study, 40 patients had FAZA-PET-CT imaging to evaluate the tracer as a prognostic factor for patients with head and neck squamous cell carcinoma undergoing radiotherapy. Twenty-two of the patients also received cisplatin.

(*purple contours*) from weeks 0 to 5 for a representative patient with early (weeks 0–2) resolution of tumor hypoxia. (*B*) Time course of tumor and hypoxic subvolumes for a representative patient with delayed (weeks 2–5) resolution of tumor hypoxia. (*From* Nicolay N, et al. Correlative analyses between tissue-based hypoxia biomarkers and hypoxia PET imaging in head and neck cancer patients during radiochemotherapy—results from a prospective trial. Eur J Nucl Med Mol Imaging. 2020;47(5):1046-1055; with permission. (Figure 3 in original).)

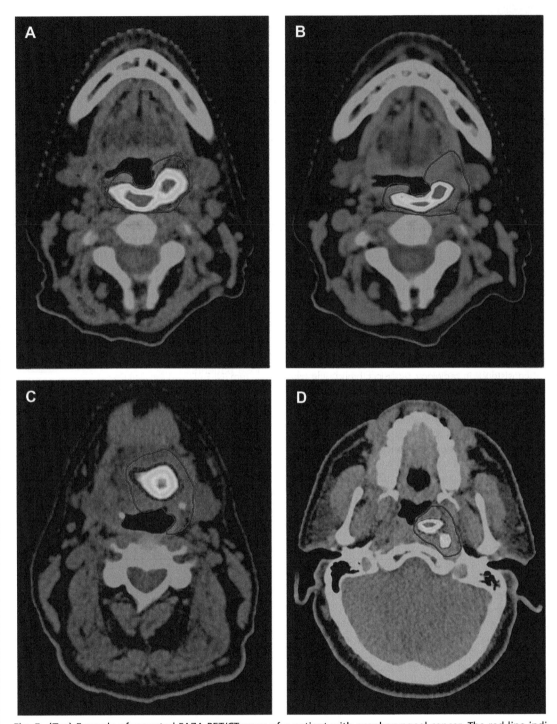

Fig. 5. (*Top*) Example of repeated FAZA-PET/CT scans of a patient with oropharyngeal cancer. The red line indicates the gross tumor volume (GTV). (*A*) The hypoxic volume (T/M ratio ≥1.4) is 30.9 cm³ at baseline. (*B*) After 12 Gy, the hypoxic volume has decreased to 13.7 cm³, but the localization remains stable. (*Bottom*) FAZA-PET/CT scans of patients with tumors having a hypoxic volume (T/M ≥ 1.4). (*C*) Male patient with an HPV-positive oropharyngeal cancer. (*D*) Male patient with an HPV-negative oropharyngeal cancer. (*From* Mortensen LS, et al. FAZA PET/CT hypoxia imaging in patients with squamous cell carcinoma of the head and neck treated with radiotherapy: Results from the DAHANCA 24 trial. Radiother Oncol. 2012;105(1):14-20; with permission. (Figure 3 in original).)

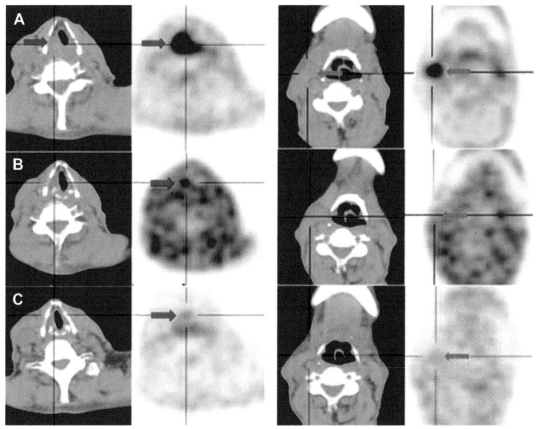

Fig. 6. A patient with hypopharyneal cancer. (*A*) Pre-FDG/CT: primary tumor (*red arrow*), lymph node metastasis (*blue arrow*). (*B*) Pre-FETNIM PET/CT: highly focally increased and visually detectable uptake in primary tumor (*red arrow*), but FETNIM uptake in lymph node metastasis similar to that of background (*blue arrow*). (*C*) Mid-FETNIM PET/CT: FETNIM uptake in primary tumor similar to that of background (*red arrow*), remains undetectable in lymph node metastasis (*blue arrow*). (*From* Hu M, et al. Hypoxia with ^{18}F-fluoroerythronitroimidazole integrated positron emission tomography and computed tomography (^{18}F-FETNIM PET/CT) in locoregionally advanced head and neck cancer: Hypoxia changes during chemoradiotherapy and impact on clinical outcome. Medicine (Baltimore). 2019;98(40):e17067; with permission. (Figure 1 in original).)

FAZA-PET imaging was performed 2 hours after injection, evaluating T/M ratios with hypoxia defined by a threshold ratio of 1.4. Hypoxia was present in 25 of 40 patients, with hypoxic tumor volumes widely varying, ranging from 0 to 30.9 mL, with no significant difference between HPV-positive and HPV-negative tumors (**Fig. 5**). After a median follow-up of 19 months, DFS was 93% in patients with nonhypoxic tumors and 60% in patients with hypoxic tumors. Thus the investigators concluded that FAZA is a suitable hypoxic imaging tracer with prognostic potential.[28]

In a prospective study, 29 patients underwent FAZA-PET-CT before treatment with chemoradiotherapy, 26 of whom had squamous cell carcinoma of the head and neck. FAZA scans started 2 hours after tracer injection. There were several significant findings in that the primary T/M ratio correlated with the primary lesion's maximum diameter; the primary T/M ratio was higher in stage 4 tumors compared with other stages; and, of all of the PET and clinical parameters that they assessed, primary T/M was the only one that significantly correlated with progression-free survival. The findings suggest that pretreatment FAZA imaging at 2 hours gives comparable imaging with FMISO imaging at 4 hours and that patients with higher FAZA measurements may benefit from more aggressive treatment because those patients with higher uptakes in the primary lesions had worse progression-free survival.[26] Another prospective study of 12 patients with locally advanced head and neck squamous cell carcinoma (stage 3 or 4) received FAZA-PET scans before and during chemoradiotherapy with repeat FAZA imaging after fractions 7 and 17 during radiotherapy. The fraction of hypoxic tumor volume decreased in

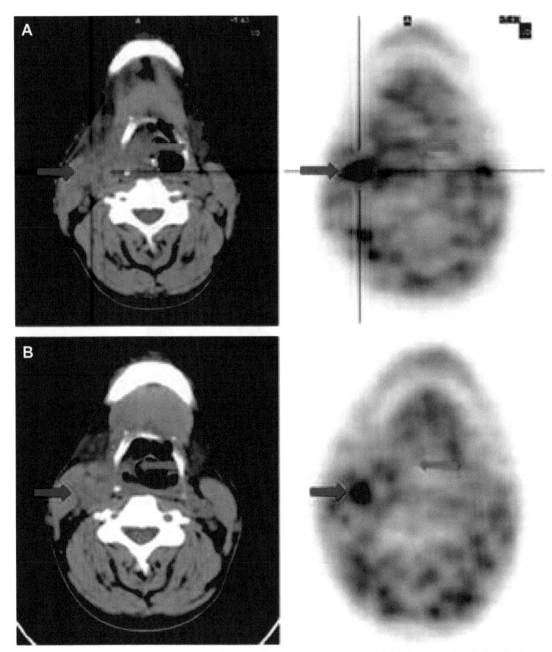

Fig. 7. Another patient with hypopharyneal cancer. (*A*) Pre-FETNIM PET/CT: highly increased and visually detectable uptake in a lymph node metastasis (*red arrow*); in contrast, FETNIM uptake in primary tumor similar to that of background (*blue arrow*). (*B*) Mid-FETNIM PET/CT: persistent FETNIM uptake in the lymph node metastasis (*red arrow*), uptake remains undetectable in primary tumor (*blue arrow*). (*From* Hu M, et al. Hypoxia with 18F-fluoroerythronitroimidazole integrated positron emission tomography and computed tomography (18F-FETNIM PET/CT) in locoregionally advanced head and neck cancer: Hypoxia changes during chemoradiotherapy and impact on clinical outcome. Medicine (Baltimore). 2019;98(40):e17067; with permission. (Figure 2 in original).)

both the primary tumor and lymph nodes throughout therapy, and, after the 17th fraction of radiotherapy, 50% of tumor and 66% of lymph nodes were no longer hypoxic and the residual hypoxic areas of tumor were less and much smaller in volume. The investigators concluded that FAZA-PET could identify and quantify hypoxic tumor volumes before and during chemoradiotherapy, and that hypoxic volumes could be identified for dose escalation, noting that repeat scans would need to be performed during treatment because of fluctuating tumor hypoxia.[27]

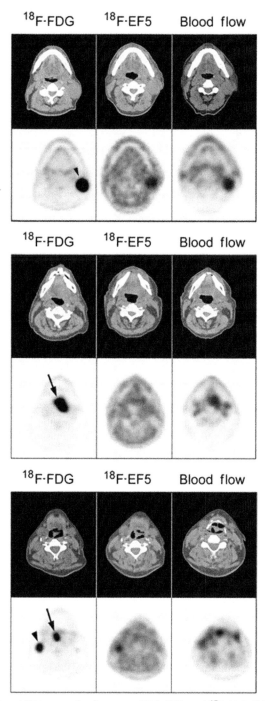

Fig. 8. Examples of both PET and CT images for 3 tracers, FDG, EF5, and ^{15}O-H_2O (blood flow) for 3 patients. EF5 images are made 3 hours after injection. Arrows indicate primary tumors, and arrowheads indicate metastatic lesions. (Komar G, Seppänen M, Eskola O, et al. 18F-EF5: a new PET tracer for imaging hypoxia in head and neck cancer. J Nucl Med 2008;49:1944-51. Figure 4. © SNMMI.)

18F-fluoroerythronitroimidazole Imaging

18F-fluoroerythronitroimidazole (FETNIM) has lower lipophilicity, like FAZA, which allows increased perfusion and blood clearance and hence faster washout from tissues that are not hypoxic with higher tumor/background ratios.[5] A recent review article states that, despite the higher tumor/background ratios of FETNIM, more work needs to be done before FETNIM can replace FMISO, FETNIM,

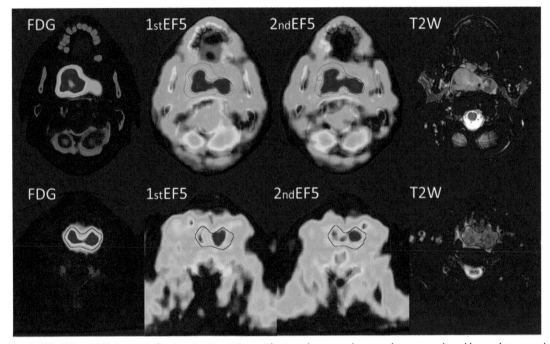

Fig. 9. PET/CT and MR images of patients presenting with nasopharyngeal cancer (*upper row*) and hypopharyngeal cancer (*lower row*). From left to right, corresponding axial slices from diagnostic FDG, the first and the second EF5-PET/CT, and fat-suppressed T2-weighted MR images are shown. The red line denotes the metabolically active tumor volume delineation using SUV 5.0 as a threshold in the FDG-PET image. The black line indicates hypoxic subvolume delineation using a T/M uptake ratio of 1.5 as a threshold in the EF5-PET image. The intrapatient voxel-by-voxel analysis showed a high correlation and agreement between the paired EF5-PET/CT images for the patient with naso-pharyngeal cancer, whereas those for the patient with hypopharyngeal cancer were among the lowest of 10 patients. (*From* Silvoniemi A, et al. Repeatability of tumour hypoxia imaging using [18F]EF5 PET/CT in head and neck cancer. Eur J Nucl Med Mol Imaging. 2018;45(2):161–169; with permission. (Figure 1 in original).)

or FAZA for hypoxic imaging.[4] However, a more recent study of 32 patients with locally advanced head and neck squamous cell carcinoma treated with chemoradiation underwent FETNIM-PET/CT before treatment and at 5 weeks of therapy. SUV-max significantly decreased in both the primary tumor and metastatic lymph nodes at 5 weeks. Both local control and overall survival were significantly worse in those patients with high pretreatment SUV-max in the primary tumor (**Fig. 6**). Distant metastatic-free survival and overall survival were both significantly worse in those patients with high SUVmax at 5 weeks (**Fig. 7**). The investigators concluded that FETNIM-PET/CT showed tumor hypoxia to significantly decrease during chemoradiation, that poor overall survival was predicated by persistent hypoxia, and that FETNIM-PET/CT could potentially be used to choose patients for hypoxia-directed treatments and aid with the appropriate timing of such treatment.[29]

18F-2-nitroimidazol-pentafluoropropyl Acetamide Imaging

18F-2-nitroimidazol-pentafluoropropyl acetamide (EF5) is also less lipophilic than FMISO, resulting in better tumor/background ratios.[4] A study

showed the potential of EF5 to detect hypoxia, when 13 primary head and neck tumors and 5 lymph nodes were evaluated at 3 hours after tracer injection with EF5-PET/CT, with comparison with FDG-PET/CT performed separately. T/M ratios more than 1.5 were noted in 14 out of 18 tumor subvolumes, indicating hypoxia[30] (**Fig. 8**). In a different study, 10 patients with untreated pharyngeal squamous cell carcinoma received 2 separate EF5-PET/CT scans a median of 7 days apart, in addition to an FDG-PET/CT scan to define the primary tumor metabolic activity. EF5-PET/CT was obtained 3 hours after injection, and a T/M ratio of 1.5 was used for the hypoxic threshold. In all 10 study pairs, good correlation was seen with SUVmean, SUVmax, and T/M ratio, and fractional hypoxic tumor volumes showed a high correlation. The investigators concluded that EF5-PET/CT scanning has high repeatability and therefore may be used to guide targeted treatment of tumor hypoxia in head and neck cancer[31] (**Fig. 9**).

18F-flortanidazole Imaging

18F-flortanidazole (HX4) also has better pharmacokinetic and clearance properties compared with FMISO, with better tumor/background ratios[5]

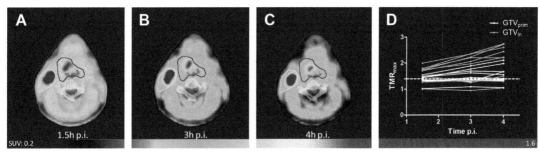

Fig. 10. HX4-PET/CT scans of a patient with a T2N2bMx squamous cell carcinoma of the oropharynx, scanned at 1.5 hours (A), 3 hours (B), and 4 hours (C) postinjection (p.i.). (D) The maximum TMR (TMR$_{max}$) for all patients. Shown are the GTVs of the primary lesions (GTV$_{prim}$) and the metastatic lymph nodes (GTV$_{ln}$), which increased significantly (1.5 hours vs 3 hours, P<.01; 3 hours vs 4 hours, P = .02). (*From* Zegers CML, et al. Evaluation of tumour hypoxia during radiotherapy using [18F] HX4 PET imaging and blood biomarkers in patients with head and neck cancer. Eur J Nucl Med Mol Imaging 2016;43(12):2139–2146; with permission. (Figure 1 in original).)

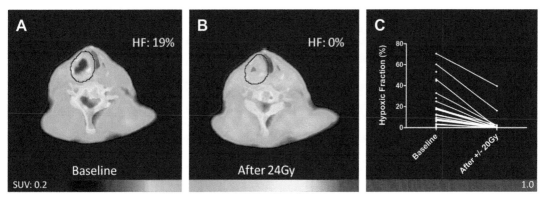

Fig. 11. HX4-PET/CT scan of a patient with a T3N2bMx squamous cell carcinoma of the hypopharynx treated with cisplatin chemoradiation. (A) Scan with hypoxic primary tumor at baseline, (B) decreased level of hypoxia during treatment, and (C) calculated hypoxic fraction (HF) of all primary tumors and lymph nodes before and during treatment, significant decrease (P<.001). (*From* Zegers CML, et al. Evaluation of tumour hypoxia during radiotherapy using [18F] HX4 PET imaging and blood biomarkers in patients with head and neck cancer. Eur J Nucl Med Mol Imaging 2016;43(12):2139–2146; with permission. (Figure 2 in original).)

(**Fig. 10**). In a study of 19 patients (9 with lung cancer and 10 with head and neck cancer), each patient received 2 serial HX4-PET/CT scans, within 1 week of each other, to examine reproducibility. SUVmax, SUVmean, tumor/background maximum, and the hypoxic tumor volume with a tumor/background ratio more than 1.2 were all significantly correlated between the 2 scans. Thus the investigators concluded that HX4-PET imaging is reproducible in the patient cohort, can be useful in assessing tumor hypoxia, and has the potential to be used for hypoxia-targeted treatments.[32] A separate study of 20 patients with head and neck cancer was performed to assess treatment-associated changes with HX4-PET/CT, hypoxic blood biomarkers, and their relation. The patients underwent HX4-PET/CT scans before treatment and again after approximately 20 Gy of radiation therapy. Hypoxia was found in 69% of

the gross tumor volumes and the hypoxic fraction significantly decreased from 21.7% to 3.6% after treatment (**Fig. 11**). Of note, the biomarkers (plasma osteopontin, carbonic anhydrase IX, and vascular endothelial growth factor) did not show significant changes during treatment. The investigators thus concluded that HX4-PET/CT can detect changes in hypoxia during treatment, whereas the blood biomarkers could not.[33]

SUMMARY

Because tumor hypoxia is an independent prognostic factor for adverse outcomes, and hypoxia subvolumes of tumor are more radiation resistant than normoxic subvolumes, much research has been performed regarding the detection of tumor hypoxia. With head and neck cancer, blood imaging biomarkers have had mixed correlations with hypoxia PET imaging tracers. Nevertheless, many studies show great clinical promise for these tracers. PET imaging is currently considered the gold standard method for imaging tumor hypoxia, with FMISO the most extensively studied hypoxic imaging tracer. Newer tracers continue to be tested that also show promise, including FAZA, FETNIM, EF5, and HX4. The current techniques show great promise for the move into the clinical realm for hypoxia, intratreatment monitoring, and the adjustment of treatment protocols with either dose escalation or dose de-escalation. Two of the main factors limiting such research are the lack of widespread availability of these tracers and the significant cost of creating them, which has essentially limited research studies thus far to smaller cohorts.

DISCLOSURE

The authors have nothing to disclose.

REFERENCES

1. Kroenke M, Hirata K, Gafita A, et al. Voxel based comparison and texture analysis of 18 F-FDG and 18 F-FMISO PET of patients with head-and-neck cancer. PLoS One 2019;14(2):1–12.
2. Swartz JE, Pothen AJ, Stegeman I, et al. Clinical implications of hypoxia biomarker expression in head and neck squamous cell carcinoma: A systematic review. Cancer Med 2015;4(7):1101–16.
3. Chirla R, Marcu LG. PET-based quantification of statistical properties of hypoxic tumor subvolumes in head and neck cancer. Phys Med 2016;32(1):23–35.
4. Marcu LG, Reid P, Bezak E. The promise of novel biomarkers for head and neck cancer from an imaging perspective. Int J Mol Sci 2018;19(9). https://doi.org/10.3390/ijms19092511.
5. Stieb S, Eleftheriou A, Warnock G, et al. Longitudinal PET imaging of tumor hypoxia during the course of radiotherapy. Eur J Nucl Med Mol Imaging 2018;45(12):2201–17.
6. Bittner MI, Wiedenmann N, Bucher S, et al. Analysis of relation between hypoxia PET imaging and tissue-based biomarkers during head and neck radiochemotherapy. Acta Oncol (Madr) 2016;55(11):1299–304.
7. Wiedenmann N, Bunea H, Rischke HC, et al. Correction to: Effect of radiochemotherapy on T2* MRI in HNSCC and its relation to FMISO PET derived hypoxia and FDG PET. Radiat Oncol 2018;13(159). https://doi.org/10.1186/s13014-018-1103-1. Radiat Oncol. 2018;13(1):1-9.
8. Sato J, Kitagawa Y, Yamazaki Y, et al. 18 F-fluoromisonidazole PET uptake is correlated with hypoxia-inducible factor-1a expression in oral squamous cell carcinoma. J Nucl Med 2013;54(7):1060–5.
9. Norikane T, Yamamoto Y, Maeda Y, et al. Correlation of 18F-fluoromisonidazole PET findings with HIF-1α and p53 expressions in head and neck cancer: Comparison with 18F-FDG PET. Nucl Med Commun 2014;35(1):30–5.
10. Okamoto S, Shiga T, Yasuda K, et al. High reproducibility of tumor hypoxia evaluated by 18F- fluoromisonidazole pet for head and neck cancer. J Nucl Med 2013;54(2):201–7.
11. Choi W, Lee SW, Park SH, et al. Planning study for available dose of hypoxic tumor volume using fluorine-18-labeled fluoromisonidazole positron emission tomography for treatment of the head and neck cancer. Radiother Oncol 2010;97(2):176–82.
12. Tamaki N, Hirata K. Tumor hypoxia: a new PET imaging biomarker in clinical oncology. Int J Clin Oncol 2016;21(4):619–25.
13. Chatterjee A, Gupta T, Rangarajan V, et al. Optimal timing of fluorine-18-fluoromisonidazole positron emission tomography/computed tomography for assessment of tumor hypoxia in patients with head and neck squamous cell carcinoma. Nucl Med Commun 2018;39(9):859–64.
14. Sato J, Kitagawa Y, Yamazaki Y, et al. Advantage of FMISO-PET over FDG-PET for predicting histological response to preoperative chemotherapy in patients with oral squamous cell carcinoma. Eur J Nucl Med Mol Imaging 2014;41(11):2031–41.
15. Sato J, Kitagawa Y, Watanabe S, et al. Hypoxic volume evaluated by 18 F-fluoromisonidazole positron emission tomography (FMISO-PET) may be a prognostic factor in patients with oral squamous cell carcinoma: preliminary analyses. Int J Oral Maxillofac Surg 2018;47(5):553–60.
16. Lee N, Schoder H, Beattie B, et al. Strategy of using intratreatment hypoxia imaging to selectively and safely guide radiation dose de-escalation concurrent with chemotherapy for locoregionally advanced human papillomavirus–related oropharyngeal carcinoma. Int J Radiat Oncol Biol Phys 2016;96(1):9–17.
17. Hendrickson K, Phillips M, Smith W, et al. Hypoxia imaging with [F-18] FMISO-PET in head and neck cancer: Potential for guiding intensity modulated radiation therapy in overcoming hypoxia-induced treatment resistance. Radiother Oncol 2011;101(3):369–75.
18. Muzi M, Krohn KA. Imaging hypoxia with 18F-fluoromisonidazole: Challenges in moving to a more complicated analysis. J Nucl Med 2016;57(4):497–8.
19. Zschaeck S, Haase R, Abolmaali N, et al. Spatial distribution of FMISO in head and neck squamous cell carcinomas during radio-chemotherapy and its

correlation to pattern of failure. Acta Oncol (Madr) 2015;54(9):1355–63.

20. Chang JH, Wada M, Anderson NJ, et al. Hypoxia-targeted radiotherapy dose painting for head and neck cancer using 18F-FMISO PET: A biological modeling study. Acta Oncol (Madr) 2013;52(8): 1723–9.

21. Toma-Dasu I, Uhrdin J, Antonovic L, et al. Dose prescription and treatment planning based on FMISO-PET hypoxia. Acta Oncol (Madr) 2012;51(2):222–30.

22. Welz S, Mönnich D, Pfannenberg C, et al. Prognostic value of dynamic hypoxia PET in head and neck cancer: Results from a planned interim analysis of a randomized phase II hypoxia-image guided dose escalation trial. Radiother Oncol 2017;124(3): 526–32.

23. Nicolay NH, Wiedenmann N, Mix M, et al. Correlative analyses between tissue-based hypoxia biomarkers and hypoxia PET imaging in head and neck cancer patients during radiochemotherapy-results from a prospective trial. Eur J Nucl Med Mol Imaging 2019. https://doi.org/10.1007/s00259-019-04598-9.

24. Löck S, Perrin R, Seidlitz A, et al. Residual tumour hypoxia in head-and-neck cancer patients undergoing primary radiochemotherapy, final results of a prospective trial on repeat FMISO-PET imaging. Radiother Oncol 2017;124(3):533–40.

25. Zips D, Zöphel K, Abolmaali N, et al. Exploratory prospective trial of hypoxia-specific PET imaging during radiochemotherapy in patients with locally advanced head-and-neck cancer. Radiother Oncol 2012;105(1):21–8.

26. Saga T, Inubushi M, Koizumi M, et al. Prognostic value of PET/CT with18F-fluoroazomycin arabinoside for patients with head and neck squamous cell carcinomas receiving chemoradiotherapy. Ann Nucl Med 2015;30(3):217–24.

27. Servagi-Vernat S, Differding S, Hanin FX, et al. A prospective clinical study of 18 F-FAZA PET-CT hypoxia imaging in head and neck squamous cell carcinoma before and during radiation therapy. Eur J Nucl Med Mol Imaging 2014;41(8):1544–52.

28. Mortensen LS, Johansen J, Kallehauge J, et al. FAZA PET/CT hypoxia imaging in patients with squamous cell carcinoma of the head and neck treated with radiotherapy: Results from the DAHANCA 24 trial. Radiother Oncol 2012;105(1):14–20.

29. Hu M, Xie P, Lee NY, et al. Hypoxia with 18F-fluoroerythronitroimidazole integrated positron emission tomography and computed tomography (18F-FETNIM PET/CT) in locoregionally advanced head and neck cancer: Hypoxia changes during chemoradiotherapy and impact on clinical outcome. Medicine (Baltimore) 2019;98(40):1–8.

30. Komar G, Seppänen M, Eskola O, et al. 18F-EF5: A new PET tracer for imaging hypoxia in head and neck cancer. J Nucl Med 2008;49(12):1944–51.

31. Silvoniemi A, Suilamo S, Laitinen T, et al. Repeatability of tumour hypoxia imaging using [18F]EF5 PET/CT in head and neck cancer. Eur J Nucl Med Mol Imaging 2018;45(2):161–9.

32. Zegers CML, van Elmpt W, Szardenings K, et al. Repeatability of hypoxia PET imaging using [18F] HX4 in lung and head and neck cancer patients: a prospective multicenter trial. Eur J Nucl Med Mol Imaging 2015;42(12):1840–9.

33. Zegers CML, Hoebers FJP, van Elmpt W, et al. Evaluation of tumour hypoxia during radiotherapy using [18F]HX4 PET imaging and blood biomarkers in patients with head and neck cancer. Eur J Nucl Med Mol Imaging 2016;43(12):2139–46.

Patient-Centric Head and Neck Cancer Radiation Therapy: Role of Advanced Imaging

Monica Shukla, MD[a], Reza Forghani, MD, PhD[b], Mohit Agarwal, MD[c],*

KEYWORDS

- Head and neck cancer • Radiation planning • Personalized • Individualized • Advanced imaging
- Functional imaging • Tumor hypoxia

KEY POINTS

- Despite the similar pathologic diagnosis, tumors differ in their behavior and response to therapy based on characteristics like cellularity, angiogenesis, tumor hypoxia and protein expression.
- To combat this heterogeneous nature of tumors, radiation therapy needs to be individualized for better outcomes.
- Advanced/functional imaging techniques and use of quantitative radiomic and machine-learning–derived biomarkers can identify areas of radioresistance by delineating unfavorable features such as hypoxia.
- Selective radiation boosts can be administered to radioresistant targets for improved treatment outcome.

INTRODUCTION

To improve disease-free and overall survival, it is imperative to understand tumor biology, which can differ across patients and even across the tumor itself. The heterogeneity of tumor cellularity and the presence of radioresistant areas (due to factors like hypoxia), which are further accentuated after initiation of therapy, emphasize the need for a more targeted, patient-centric treatment, that can allow intratreatment adaptation of initial treatment plan, such as dose escalation to poorly responding areas. Histopathological evaluation of tumor heterogeneity by biopsy of different tumor regions is not feasible, but increasingly, sophisticated advanced imaging techniques can serve as noninvasive biomarkers that can delineate tumor hypoxia, cellularity, vascularity, and even tumor molecular profile. In this article, we discuss these advanced imaging modalities and provide a general outline of the current approach in patient-centric radiation treatment.

OVERVIEW OF HEAD AND NECK CANCER AND RADIATION TREATMENT

Head and neck cancers (HNCs) are a varied group of malignancies that comprise approximately 7% of all new cancers diagnosed in the United States per year, and taken together, the fourth most common group of cancers worldwide.[1,2] Despite many advancements in diagnosis and treatment, taken as a group, 5-year overall survival (OS) hovers at approximately 60%.[2,3]

Traditional risk factors for HNCs have been tobacco and alcohol use, particularly for squamous cell carcinoma arising from epithelial lining of upper aerodigestive tract. However, the epidemiology for

[a] Department of Radiation Oncology, Froedtert and Medical College of Wisconsin, 9200 W. Wisconsin Avenue, Milwaukee, WI 53226, USA; [b] Augmented Intelligence & Precision Health Laboratory, Department of Radiology, Research Institute of McGill University Health Centre, 1001 Decarie Boulevard, Montreal, Quebec H4A 3J1, Canada; [c] Department of Radiology, Section of Neuroradiology, Froedtert and Medical College of Wisconsin, 8701 Watertown Plank Road, Milwaukee, WI 53226, USA

* Corresponding author.
E-mail address: magarwal@mcw.edu

Neuroimag Clin N Am 30 (2020) 341–357
https://doi.org/10.1016/j.nic.2020.04.005

oropharyngeal cancers, in particular, has shifted in the past several decades, with declining smoking rates and increased incidence of cancers associated with the human papilloma virus, which vastly differ in biology and prognosis,[3] so much so, that they are now regarded as a separate entity in the eighth edition of the American Joint Committee on Cancer staging manual.[4] Similarly, a separate system has been developed for Epstein-Barr virus–associated nasopharyngeal cancers. Traditionally, surgery has been the primary therapy, with radiation therapy (RT) used postoperatively to eradicate any microscopic residual disease. In the 1980s, the organ preservation paradigm took hold, bringing in the use of RT as a definitive treatment modality. Later, combined with chemotherapy, further improvements were seen in locoregional cancer control and organ preservation rates, albeit at the cost of increased toxicity.[5,6]

RT is still used postoperatively in patients with locally advanced tumors and intermediate-risk pathologic features, such as perineural invasion, lymphovascular invasion, poor differentiation, and multiple involved lymph nodes.[7] Concurrent chemotherapy is added in patients with positive margins or extracapsular nodal extension to improve locoregional control (LRC), disease-free survival, and OS.[8]

Close proximity of head and neck to critical and sensitive organs makes it challenging to treat with RT. With the advent of highly conformal RT, namely intensity-modulated RT or IMRT, RT can be delivered precisely to the tumor, while sparing surrounding normal structures. IMRT has significantly improved the therapeutic ratio in the curative intent setting and allowed for increased use in the salvage setting in prior irradiated fields in which sparing of organs at risk (OARs) carries even more importance. Also increasing in use is stereotactic body RT (SBRT), which is used as a definitive modality for individuals who are not candidates for a long, aggressive course of concurrent chemoradiotherapy or those with a new primary tumor or a recurrence in a prior irradiated field.[9] Advantages of SBRT are the high conformality of the delivered dose, high dose per treatment (which is considered to be more biologically effective), and the fact that it is delivered over a much shorter period (generally 5 sessions over 1.5–2.0 weeks), which is particularly important in a frail population. The high dose per treatment, however, can be more destructive to the surrounding normal tissue,[10] thus precision with treatment setup and definition of treatment volumes and adherence to predefined normal tissue dose constraints is of utmost importance.

Traditional radiation dose and fractionation for HNC has used a "one-size-fits-all approach." Total doses range from 50 to 70 Gy, depending on the setting. Doses are often reduced around critical OARs (eg, optic nerves, brain stem, spinal cord) in cases with high risk-to-benefit ratio.

A momentous study published by Scott and colleagues[11] in 2017 took some of the first steps in creating a model that could be used as a basis to tailor RT dose to individual tumor radiosensitivity. Although this is transformative work, we know that there is significant geographic intratumoral variation in terms of gene expression. Thus, a tissue sample taken from one area of a tumor may not be representative of another. If one were looking to tailor RT to an individual tumor, it is possible that different parts of the tumor may require different doses of RT to achieve a cure. It is also possible that different areas of the tumor would respond better to RT delivered differently with regard to dose per fraction, total treatment time, or perhaps delivered in concert with systemic therapy (chemotherapy or immunotherapy). Another point to consider is that the tumor biology may change significantly during the standard 6 to 7 weeks of RT. This provides opportunity for treatment-intensity escalation to areas of tumor responding sluggishly to treatment while deescalation of therapy to those areas responding well.

Although geographic and temporal intra-tumoral genotypic expression variations are ripe for use for personalized radiation, it is not feasible to biopsy as many areas in a tumor as would be desired or with acceptable frequency. This is where tailoring therapy based on imaging biomarkers provides an opportunity. In this regard, the growing field of computerized image analysis and radiomics enabling extraction of high-level quantitative information from both standard and advanced imaging techniques to better characterize the biological phenotype of each individual tumor and predict clinical tumor behavior has great potential,[12,13] as is discussed later in this article.

RADIATION TREATMENT PLANNING

Currently computed tomography (CT), most often with contrast, is used for segmentation of both normal structures (OARs) as well as treatment volumes, although practices can vary across institutions. IMRT and variations thereof, such as volumetric arc modulated therapy and helical tomotherapy, is the standard technique used for creation of definitive and postoperative head and neck RT plans. The patient is positioned on the treatment table with the help of on-board imaging with either kV or mV cone beam CT or kV CT-on-rails, which is used to confirm accurate daily set up. Significant changes in both the tumor volume and general dimensions of the patient and OARs that occur as a result of therapy can be noted. MR imaging is also being used for target delineation and daily treatment modification.[14] Daily onboard 3-dimensional imaging allows monitoring of changes and adaptation of the RT plan, thus preventing underdosing of target volumes and overdosing of normal structures. Some treatment machines with their proprietary software allow for online adaptation of treatment (while the patient is on the treatment table), although the vast majority of centers at this time perform offline adaptation.[15]

As mentioned earlier, current standard treatment planning and delivery are largely based on traditional approaches using limited anatomic information and precludes many of the advanced imaging techniques or emerging quantitative image biomarkers, such as radiomics, that may enable more precise and personalized therapy. This is likely to change in the future. In the following sections, we discuss the various advanced and functional imaging techniques that allow radiologists/radiation oncologists to visualize various characteristics within a tumor, such as proliferation and perfusion, and how they can and have been used to personalize RT.

PERFUSION MR IMAGING

Neoangiogenesis, or formation of new vessels, is a feature of malignant processes. These new vessels, however, are marked by tortuosity, increased density, poor functionality, and higher permeability,[16–18] which alters the vascular properties of malignant tissue.[18] This feature is used in the differentiation and assessment of tumors in perfusion imaging.[19,20] Three types of perfusion MR imaging are in practice, namely, dynamic contrast enhanced (DCE) MR imaging, dynamic susceptibility contrast (DSC) MR imaging, and arterial spin labeling (ASL) MR imaging.[16,21] The quality and usability of DSC and ASL-MR imaging is limited in the head and neck due to susceptibility artifacts produced by the many air-tissue interfaces. From a practical standpoint, DCE-MR imaging is the most useable and is therefore more popular than DSC-MR imaging or ASL (Fig. 1).

In DCE-MR imaging, rapid sequential T1-weighted MR images are obtained before, during, and after the administration of gadolinium-based contrast agent. This quantitative assessment involves 3 basic steps: acquisition of precontrast baseline T1 map, acquisition of dynamic data during the administration of contrast, and finally the assessment of arterial input function (AIF). AIF is determined by placing a region of interest over a visible artery in the dynamic dataset and obtaining

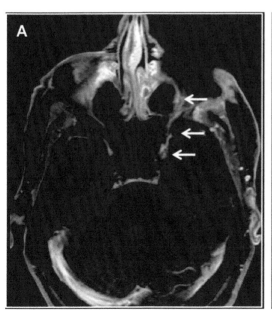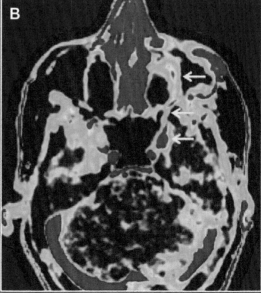

Fig. 1. Axial postcontrast T1-weighted fat-suppressed MR imaging image (A) in a patient with orbital squamous cell carcinoma shows subtle enhancement along infraorbital nerve and V2 (white arrows). AUC DCE perfusion MR imaging map (B) demonstrates the perineural spread much more clearly (yellow arrows). (Courtesy of A. Srinivasan, MD, University of Michigan, Ann Arbor.)

data on the enhancement kinetics of the artery perfusing the area of interest. Standard pharmacokinetic parameters based on the kinetics of the contrast agent concentration within the vascular space and extravascular extracellular space (EES) are then calculated; which include K_{trans} (the transfer rate constant for contrast from the plasma into the EES), K_{ep} (rate constant from the EES to the vascular space), V_e (volume of the EES per unit volume of tissue), PS (permeability surface area product per unit of mass of tissue), F (flow of whole blood per unit mass of tissue), and V_p (fractional plasma volume). Semiquantitative analysis can also be done, where the derived time intensity curves are used to demonstrate parameters such as wash-in slope, time to peak enhancement, maximum peak enhancement, wash-out slope, and area under the curve (AUC)[21–25] (**Fig. 2**).

The technique allows a visual correlate of tumor blood flow, which is a potential surrogate for local vascular permeability, oxygen distribution, and pH.[26,27] The aforementioned neoangiogenesis, characterized by dysfunctional vessels, results in

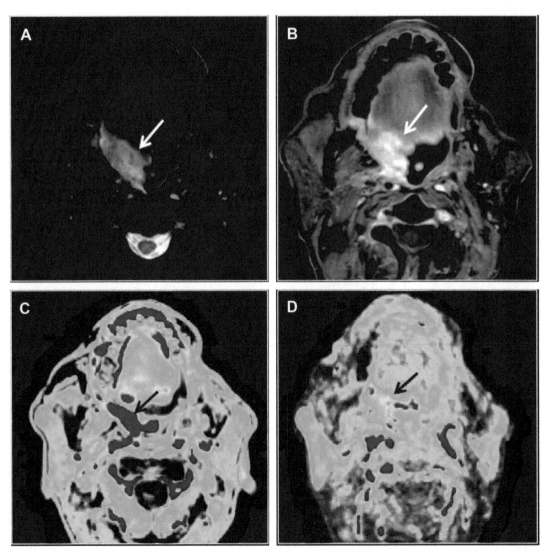

Fig. 2. Axial short tau inversion recovery (STIR) (*A*) and axial postcontrast fat-suppressed T1-weighted MR images (*B*) in a patient with a history of right tongue base squamous cell carcinoma. Posttreatment change and recurrent tumor are difficult to distinguish amidst the STIR hyperintense signal in the treatment bed (*arrow* in *A*) and postcontrast enhancement (*arrow* in *B*). Total plasma volume (Vp) DCE-MR image (*C*) and Ktrans DCE_MR image (*D*) better delineate the recurrent tumor (*black arrows*). (*Courtesy of* A. Srinivasan, MD, University of Michigan, Ann Arbor.)

hypoperfusion and development of areas of hypoxia.[18] These hypoxic areas are generally felt to be radioresistant and clinically have been correlated with poorer LRC.[28,29] There is evidence in vitro and in vivo that a significantly increased dose of RT (in the range of 2–3 times more) is needed to overcome the radioresistance conferred by hypoxia.[20,29,30]

The most widely investigated parameters in DCE-MR imaging are K_{trans} and V_e. Newbold and colleagues[26,31] have shown that tumors with high K_{trans} and V_e had low fractions of tumor hypoxia. Another study, by Donaldson and colleagues,[32] found that tumors with increased hypoxic tissue had lower values of perfusion. Higher pretreatment values have been associated with improved outcomes and better OS in a study by Jensen and colleagues.[33] Hoskin and colleagues[34] showed a correlation between level of maximum enhancement on DCE-MR imaging and improved LRC. Another review highlighted several studies that were successful in correlating imaging findings to at least short-term cancer outcomes.[35]

DCE-MR imaging can also be used to reflect treatment response (TtR) after RT, where higher blood volume and blood flow are seen in patients with complete response.[17,36] The ability of DCE-MR imaging to assess TtR can be used in intratreatment evaluation for predicting outcome. Wang and colleagues[36] showed that low perfusion metrics 2 weeks after initiation of treatment were predictive of local treatment failure.[19] Evaluation of tumor perfusion early on during the course of the treatment and demonstration of low perfusion parameters (which are correlated with tumor hypoxia) can also steer the treatment toward dose

intensification and help in individualized therapy.[19,21,28,37–48]

DIFFUSION-WEIGHTED IMAGING

Diffusion-weighted MR imaging (DWI) is based on molecular diffusion of protons corresponding to Brownian motion and can reflect underlying tissue microstructure and cellularity based on apparent diffusion coefficient (ADC) maps,[49] where lower ADC values are correlated with higher cellularity.[22,49,50]

DWI can be used for characterization of primary tumors, with malignant lymphoma demonstrating relatively lower ADC values among all tumors.[51–53] ADC values have been found to be a strong predictor for the presence of nodal metastasis and detection of small metastatic nodes is greatly improved by DWI.[54,55] Conflicting reports are available for prognostic values of pretreatment ADC, which could be due to the heterogeneity of techniques and MR scanners across different sites, but in most studies high pretreatment ADC is known to be associated with poor prognostic outcome.[56,57] High stromal content, low cellularity, micronecrosis, and p16 negativity are associated with poor TtR and prognosis, and these characteristics are associated with higher ADC.[53,58–60]

DWI also has been reported to help in differentiating between tumor and post-RT changes,[43,56,61–67] (Fig. 3), immediately after RT and has been shown to be of greater specificity compared with fludeoxyglucose (FDG)-PET in this period.[68] Because further therapy can be tailored to the individual patient, the determination of TtR becomes important.[69] Intratreatment monitoring of ADC values during RT has proven useful

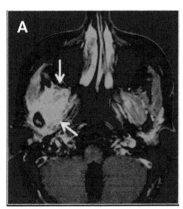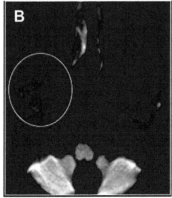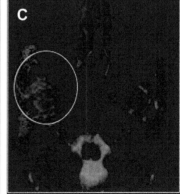

Fig. 3. Axial postcontrast fat-suppressed T1-weighted MR image (*A*) shows avid enhancement in the right masticator space (*arrows*) concerning for recurrent tumor. Axial DWI (*B*) and ADC (*C*) images show no associated restricted diffusion (*circles*). Granulation tissue was found at biopsy. (*Courtesy of* A. Srinivasan, MD, University of Michigan, Ann Arbor.)

in some studies, with evidence that a lower increase or decrease in ADC values 1 to 4 weeks into RT are more likely to fail treatment.[43,63,65] Studies suggest that a smaller percentage rise (lower fractional change) in the mean ADC values within the first to third weeks of treatment is associated with poor treatment outcome.[22,43,61–65] The assessment of fractional change may be of benefit in circumventing the heterogeneity produced by different techniques and scanners across different sites.[69] Quantitative diffusion metrics can also distinguish residual/recurrent tumor tissue from posttreatment changes, in which residual/recurrent disease demonstrates lower ADC values compared with benign posttreatment tissue.[56]

More recently, monoexponential and biexponential models are being used for quantification of diffusion. The diffusion sensitizing effects from the encoding gradients are indicated by the b-value. The low b-value diffusion images reflect microvascularity and tissue perfusion because fast-moving water molecules quickly lose their phase even at low values. High b-value images represent tissue cellularity. Monoexponential ADC values cannot separate pure molecular diffusion from motion of water molecules in the capillary network. Multiexponential models that use several b-values offer more accurate quantification of diffusion without perfusion contamination.[70–73] Intravoxel incoherent motion (IVIM) and diffusion kurtosis imaging use these multiexponential models and present more accurate evaluation of the diffusion metrics.[70] Several new and unique diffusion metrics, such as pure molecular diffusion (D), perfusion-related diffusion (D*), and perfusion fraction (f), can be calculated by IVIM. The D values are higher in tumors that show poor TtR. Intratreatment IVIM studies show that tumors exhibiting higher D values and larger percent reductions in (f) were associated with locoregional failure.[69,74] The evaluation of fractional change, that is, percentage change, may again be of value in avoiding the problems posed by scanner and technique differences.

More refined analysis of DWI data has also been studied, which creates possibilities for personalized intratreatment dose modification targeting cellular changes. In a study by Galban and colleagues,[75] a voxel-wise approach was used for the evaluation of ADC changes during treatment that involves calculation of parametric response maps, which may be more sensitive to cellular changes than change in the mean ADC over the whole area of interest.[19,45] This provides opportunity for dose painting, a form of personalized treatment that is discussed in greater detail later in this article.

BLOOD OXYGEN LEVEL–DEPENDENT MR IMAGING

Blood oxygen level–dependent (BOLD) MR imaging is an imaging technique that can serve to identify areas of tumor hypoxia. Paramagnetic properties of deoxyhemoglobin in red blood cells are exploited to create contrast in this technique. Deoxyhemoglobin causes magnetic susceptibility alterations that produce changes in T2*-weighted images. Transverse MR relaxation rate R2*, which is the inverse of T2*(1/T2*) is a sensitive index of tissue oxygenation and can be used to map areas of tumor hypoxia. Baseline R2* has been found to be an independent prognostic factor for patient survival, and lower baseline R2* values are associated with increased TtR.[19,76–78]

MR SPECTROSCOPY

MR spectroscopy (MRS) is a noninvasive method that allows measurement of metabolite concentration and has the potential to determine metabolic changes in the tissues affected by cancer. The different metabolite resonances that have been used in tumor imaging are choline (Ch), creatine (Cr), lactate, and lipid.[79] Choline is a marker of membrane biosynthesis and reflects cellular proliferation. Creatine is used as an internal reference for measuring changes in other metabolites because it serves as a reservoir for high-energy phosphates, and cellular energy is typically maintained at a constant level.[79] Increased lipid and lactate within tissues are associated with hypoxic and necrotic regions. MRS may thus be used as another technique to determine tumor hypoxia.[79–81]

PERFUSION COMPUTED TOMOGRAPHY

Continuous recording of X-ray attenuation over an area of interest is done during passage of a bolus of iodinated contrast medium in this technique. The dynamic acquisition allows generation of time-attenuation curves by the use of a deconvolution algorithm. Perfusion parameters, such as blood flow (BF), blood volume (BV), mean transit time (MTT), and capillary permeability, are derived. The technique may allow differentiation of malignant from nonmalignant lesions, with malignant lesions showing a shorter time to peak/MTT and increased BF and BV. The ability of this technique to detect tissue vascularity also can be used to differentiate recurrent tumors from posttreatment changes, where recurrent disease is associated with higher CT perfusion parameters.[17,21,38,44,82]

Microvessel density (MVD) is a pathologic marker of neoangiogenesis. MVD can be evaluated noninvasively by CT perfusion and forms an important constituent of the functional imaging arsenal to image tumor hypoxia. Increased MVD, which implies increased tumor hypoxia, is associated with an increased risk of locoregional recurrence and decreased survival.[82]

DUAL-ENERGY COMPUTED TOMOGRAPHY

Dual-energy CT (DECT) is reviewed in greater detail in the Thiparom Sananmuang and colleagues' article, "Dual Energy CT in Head and Neck Imaging: Pushing the Envelope," elsewhere in this issue, and therefore will only be briefly discussed here. DECT uses the advantages offered by the use of 2 X-ray spectra, instead of the one used in the usual single-energy scans (SECTs), which allows material characterization and differentiation beyond what is done with SECT.[83–86] In addition to enabling reconstruction of images similar to a standard SECT, DECT can be used to generate reconstructions not possible with SECT. One example is the virtual monochromatic image (VMI). In this type of reconstruction, the data from the 2 different spectra can be combined in different ways to create images simulating a CT acquisition (1) as if it were obtained using a pure monochromatic beam (which is not done in clinical scanners in which a polychromatic beam is used for practical and technical feasibility reasons), and (2) at a wide range of prescribed or predetermined energies that can then be exploited to enhance diagnostic interpretation and tumor characterization. Another type of reconstruction unique to DECT is the basis material decomposition map. Using this approach, for certain materials, DECT can be used to create a map representing the relative distribution and concentration of the materials. Different types of maps have described in the literature, but from a head and neck oncology perspective, one that is of interest is the iodine map, reflecting the distribution and estimated iodine content within the tumor, which in turn is reflective of tumor vascularity.

Using VMIs and/or iodine material decomposition maps, one of the most important roles of DECT in treatment panning could be accurate delineation of tumor margins, including invasion of critical organs, such as thyroid cartilage, and possibly improving detection of metastatic lymphadenopathy. Low-energy VMI reconstructions have been reported to improve tumor visibility and margin discrimination in several research studies,[87–92] and therefore could play an important role in the determination of tumor volumes for therapy planning. Low-energy VMIs and quantitative spectral Hounsfield unit curve analysis also may

be used to enhance the detection of metastatic lymph nodes.[88,90] Furthermore, low-energy VMIs have not only be shown to improve tumor visibility in untreated tumors, these reconstructions in addition to iodine maps also have been shown to have utility in the posttreatment neck for improving detection and discrimination of posttreatment changes from recurrent tumor.[89,93–96] For evaluation of critical organ invasion, such as the thyroid cartilage, studies have also reported the usefulness of DECT in the determination of thyroid cartilage invasion (Fig. 4). On high-energy VMIs, there is relative preservation of the attenuation of the cartilage, but relative decrease of tumor attenuation, allowing for distinction of tumor from the cartilage.[97] Iodine maps have also been shown to be useful for improving accuracy of thyroid cartilage invasion.[97–99] These all represent opportunities for more precise, personalized therapy. Indeed, early studies suggest that quantitative features derived from DECT scans can help predict locoregional recurrence in HNC.[100]

At a more general level, in addition to a degree of inherent artifact reduction by simulating a monochromatic beam acquisition, high-energy VMIs have also shown utility for metal artifact reduction in individuals with dental implants, prosthetic material, and similar objects causing image degradation, although for dental artifact the results are variable and modest at best, and at the expense of decreased soft tissue contrast and reduction in iodine attenuation within enhancing tumor.[101] More specific to radiation oncology, DECT has also proven useful in radiation dose calculation and treatment planning. When a greater number of high-density and high atomic number structures are in the planning field, DECT-derived calculations show more accurate and reliable inhomogeneity corrections. For example, Hudobivnik and colleagues[102] compared the proton therapy treatment planning of tumors at the skull base to calculate the stopping powers while using SECT and DECT, and confirmed a higher accuracy for DECT in their surrogate patients using a pencil beam algorithm. Last, as is discussed in the section on radiomics and artificial intelligence (AI), there are emerging examples that the rich quantitative data from DECT scans can be leveraged for improved biomarker development.

PET WITH FLUOXYGLUCOSE F 18

Increased metabolic activity and glucose utilization by malignant cells is exploited by PET with FDG F18 (^{18}F FDG-PET) imaging, which is an integral part of pretreatment planning for head and neck tumors. Accounting for nonspecific nature

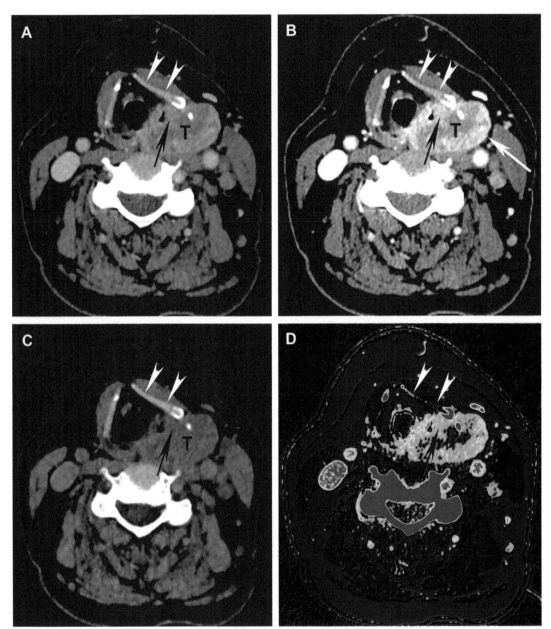

Fig. 4. Different DECT reconstructions and applications for tumor boundary delineation and distinction of non-ossified thyroid cartilage from tumor. (*A*) 65 keV VMI, (*B*) 40 keV VMI, (*C*) 140 keV VMI, and (*D*) iodine-water (IW) map reconstructed from the same infused DECT examination demonstrate a large heterogeneously enhancing hypopharyngeal mass (T). There is increased attenuation and improved delineation of tumor–soft tissue boundaries on the 40 keV compared with 65 keV VMI. In addition, a small part of the tumor extends adjacent to the left thyroid cartilage that is mostly nonossified. Note how nonossified thyroid cartilage (*arrowheads*) has attenuation close to that of enhancing tumor on 65 or 40 keV VMIs (*black arrow*). However, on the 140 keV VMI, there is suppression of tumor attenuation but relative preservation of nonossified thyroid cartilage attenuation that clearly is higher and distinguishable from tumor. On the IW map, the tumor margins are well delineated and there is absence of iodine signal within intact nonossified thyroid cartilage. Of note, there is a heterogeneously enhancing pathologic left level III lymph node. The *white arrow* in (*B*) denotes the non-ossified tumor extending adjacent to the left thyroid cartilage.

of the tracer uptake, ^{18}F FDG-PET scans often reveal tumor tissue, lymph node spread, and distant metastasis not discovered by other imaging modalities. Many radiologists continue to rely on maximum standardized uptake (SUV_{max})values for differentiation of malignant tissue, but studies have shown that the cutoff values and related sensitivities and specificities differ widely, so that no single value has emerged as a universal cutoff.[80,103]

^{18}F FDG-PET has been found to be of considerable use in the delineation of gross tumor volume[104,105] (**Fig. 5**). The low spatial resolution of PET, however, makes this a challenging task. Automated segmentation methods offer an advantage in this regard. Several such methods are in use, without a single one proven to match the exact tumor volume.[80,106,107] The gradient-based method developed by Geets and colleagues,[108] which aimed at improved image quality by denoising and deblurring, showed that it provided a better estimate of true tumor volume compared with other conventional threshold-based approaches.

^{18}F FDG-PET can be integrated in IMRT planning and has been proven to be beneficial for treatment personalization and dose escalation.

Castadot and colleagues[109] performed ^{18}F FDG-PET scans before and during therapy and found that there was change not only in tumor volume but also in the position of target volumes and OARs. This change motivates adaptive strategies, whereby dose modification can be done depending on the new tumor status. An important concept in this realm is that of "dose painting." Dose painting involves the delivery of a higher dose to an additional PET-based target volume inside the tumor. A uniform dose is prescribed for target subvolumes in "dose painting by contours" and a voxel-wise heterogeneous dose derived from the various subvolume uptake levels is prescribed in "dose painting by numbers."[40,80,110–113]

HYPOXIA PET IMAGING

Hypoxia confers radioresistance on the tumor and alters the tumor biology by stimulating angiogenesis. To improve outcomes of therapy, hypoxia modification methods, such as accelerated RT with carbogen and nicotinamide and the hypoxic sensitizer nimorazole, have been used. Although hypoxic areas can be detected by histologic markers, imaging evaluation of hypoxic areas in

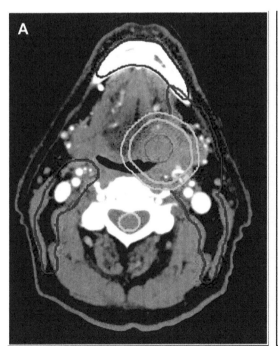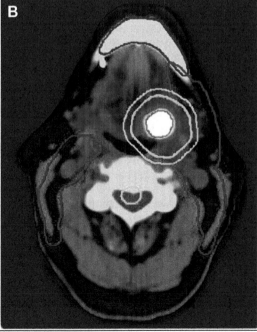

Fig. 5. Axial CT with contrast (*A*) done in the RT treatment planning position (simulation scan) and a registered diagnostic PET/CT scan (*B*) of the same patient (73-year-old man with cT2N0M0 p16+ tumor). It is difficult to define the extent of this base of tongue/glossotonsillar sulcus lesion on the planning CT alone. As is shown, the PET/CT scan aids significantly in defining the position, shape and border of this tumor. This patient was treated to a total dose of 66 Gy in 30 fx, RT alone. PTV 66 Gy is shown in green, PTV 60 Gy in gold and PTV 54 Gy in red.

the tumor is desirable due to heterogeneity of distribution of hypoxic areas within the tumor and because imaging offers the advantage of mapping the entire extent of the tumor.[17,26,38,80,114,115]

Nitroimidazole-based compounds, such as misonidazole and pimonidazole, selectively bind to hypoxic cells and can be used as PET tracers of hypoxia. The 2 best-known tracers are ^{18}F-fluoromisonidazole (^{18}F-FMISO) and ^{18}F-fluoroazomycin arabinoside (^{18}F-FAZA). High levels of hypoxia shown by ^{18}F-FMISO are associated with locoregional treatment failure.[26,80,113,116,117] A stronger prognostic value was found with intratreatment early imaging allowing for dose escalation and introduction of hypoxia modifiers.[118] An interesting and important phenomenon is that hypoxic regions may fluctuate during treatment. This requires consideration of active personalized intervention based on hypoxic tumor volumes. Tumor reoxygenation may also occur, which creates an interesting picture of dynamically altering regions of tumor hypoxia and reoxygenation, in which a voxel-wise dose painting by numbers based on hypoxia PET intuitively seems to be of benefit.[119]

CELL PROLIFERATION PET IMAGING

Tumors showing a successful response to therapy have been shown to demonstrate rapid decrease in cell proliferation. On the other hand, posttreatment compensatory tumor cell proliferative activity have been seen to impact outcomes in an adverse manner.[17,120–122] Increased DNA synthesis during enhanced cell proliferation leads to increased activity of an enzyme thymidine kinase 1 (TK1), which is involved in incorporation of the nucleoside thymidine into the DNA. Thymidine analogue 3'-deoxy-3'-[^{18}F] fluorothymidine (^{18}F-FLT) can be used as a PET tracer exploiting the activity of TK1 as a surrogate biomarker for increased cell proliferation.[118,120,121]

It has been shown in studies that ^{18}F-FLT can detect changes in tumor metabolism early on, even before the tumor shows change in volume or morphology. In Hoeben and colleagues,[118,123] the decrease in SUV_{max} between scans performed at baseline and the second week predicted a better 3-year disease-free survival. On the other hand, in a study by Troost and colleagues,[104] high proliferative tumor subvolumes detected by ^{18}F-FLT motivated an IMRT plan with dose escalation in these regions. Repeated ^{18}F-FLT PET during treatment has thus been correlated with favorable outcomes due to the facilitation of active patient-centric intervention based on changes in tumor biology early on.[26,80,117] The cell proliferation

noted with tumors is not a feature of posttreatment inflammation, which increases the specificity of ^{18}F-FLT PET and makes it more valuable in intratreatment and posttreatment monitoring and in the development of personalized therapy.[124]

ANGIOGENESIS PET AND IMMUNO-PET IMAGING

Availability and demonstrated benefit of antiangiogenic drugs targeted against angiogenic factors highlights the need for imaging modalities that can detect tumor neoangionenesis.[125] ^{18}F-Galacto-RGD PET is a promising tracer that binds to angiogenesis molecular targets, such as avß3 integrins, and helps in detecting tumor angiogenesis.[126] ^{18}F-Galacto-RGD PET has been found to be sensitive enough to visualize avß3 expression resulting exclusively from tumor vasculature and enables noninvasive quantitative assessment of avß3 expression pattern on tumor and endothelial cells.[127,128] In a study by Chen and colleagues,[129] the uptake of ^{18}F-Galacto-RGD was significantly lower in those who achieved complete response than in those with residual tumors. With further development of this technique, ^{18}F-Galacto-RGD PET can be used in tumor response monitoring and individualized radiation planning.

Immunologic markers such as antibodies, antibody fragments, and molecule inhibitors can be tagged using specific PET tracers and can be used in mapping protein expression, adding prognostic value.[118] In a study by Li and colleagues,[130] a PET tracer 18F-FBEM was used for tagging epidermal growth factor receptor (EGFR) in head and neck squamous cell carcinoma UM-SCC1 cell line. Higher uptake was seen in EGFR-positive tumors, which confers radioresistance and predicts unfavorable outcome. Studies are under way for development of tracers specific to other molecular markers, such as KRAS, C-MET, and TP53.[131]

SINGLE-PHOTON EMISSION COMPUTED TOMOGRAPHY

The three-dimensional image produced by single-photon emission CT (SPECT) imaging offers advantages of improved assessment; however, the reduced spatial resolution compared with PET limits its clinical use. Carbonic anhydrase IX (CAIX) is an enzyme expressed on the surface of the tumor cells and plays a key role in the adaptation of tumor cells to hypoxia. The tumor cells upregulate the expression of CAIX under hypoxic conditions. Noninvasive imaging detection of CAIX expression can be used to identify tumor hypoxia. Recently, an SPECT tracer [^{111}In] In-DTPA-girentuximab-F(ab')$_2$ has been developed for imaging evaluation of CAIX. This opens up another avenue for intratreatment tumor hypoxia imaging and individualized treatment modulation.[132,133]

RADIOMICS AND ARTIFICIAL INTELLIGENCE

It is likely that radiomics and AI, especially (but not solely) the machine learning subfield of AI, will play an important role in future diagnosis and patient-centric treatment of HNCs. Radiomics is a rapidly developing field in the world of medical imaging based on evidence that quantitative information can be extracted from clinical images and that this information is a reflection of underlying pathophysiology, tumor biology, and genetics, serving as a noninvasive biomarker. First introduced in the literature in 2012, radiomics was initially defined as the high-throughput extraction of large amounts of image features from radiographic images, and the definition subsequently expanded to include the conversion of images to higher dimensional data and the subsequent mining of these data for improved clinical decision support.[134–137] This quantitative information has the potential to reveal unique characteristics of individual tumors and patients and pave the way for personalized treatment.

Radiomic features can be hand-crafted (or hand-engineered), meaning that the features were designed by experts using predefined mathematical or algebraic formulas, or deep, meaning that they were extracted based on analysis of data using deep learning, a type of machine learning. In addition to enabling extraction of deep features, various machine-learning approaches, including but not limited to deep learning, also have the potential to generate prediction models serving as noninvasive biomarkers for personalized cancer therapy. When combined, these approaches have the potential to better leverage existing quantitative information on a patient's conventional or advanced imaging scans to derive otherwise unknown tumor biomarkers that enhance diagnostic evaluation and prediction of tumor biologic behavior, response to treatment, and even prediction of certain molecular phenotypes.[136,138,139] Interestingly, as alluded to earlier, the large amount of quantitative information available on a DECT scan may also be leveraged to enhance tumor characterization and biomarker development,[140,141] an area of increasing interest and future research. One example of application of radiomics is the use of radiomic features to map tumor heterogeneity more precisely, which enables voxel-wise analysis of the tumors and allows individualization of radiation planning by selective dosing. A greater and more specific discussion of these interesting topics, including the many examples of head and neck–specific applications of radiomics and a broader discussion of the role of computerized image analysis and AI, including for automated contouring and streamlining RT and adaptive planning, are beyond the scope of this article.

SUMMARY

In this era of individualized patient-centric treatment, advanced imaging techniques can make an impact on outcome by more precise estimation of tumor volume and improved delineation of the tumor margins. Detection of adjacent structure involvement and recognition of occult locoregional metastasis made possible by advanced imaging can aid in more accurate staging of the tumor. Functional imaging techniques, such as DCE, MRS, BOLD, and PET, can help determine radio-resistant regions due to hypoxia or accelerated proliferation and move the treatment toward dose escalation by techniques such as IMRT boosts. The availability of these advanced methods and the ability to delineate tumor heterogeneity combined with cutting-edge techniques, like radiomics and machine learning, facilitate identification of targets for voxel-wise selective radiation boosts and have caused a paradigm shift in RT, which has moved away from the "one-size-fits-all" approach and is increasingly tailored to individualized treatment.

ACKNOWLEDGMENTS

The authors express their sincere gratitude to Prof. Ashok Srinivasan of University of Michigan for contributing images to this article.

DISCLOSURE

R. Forghani has acted as speaker and consultant for GE Healthcare and has a research agreement (beta tester) and research support from GE Healthcare. R. Forghani is also a founder and stockholder of 4intelligent Inc.

REFERENCES

1. National Comprehensive Cancer Network. Head Neck Cancer 2019;3.
2. Bray F, Ferlay J, Soerjomataram I, et al. Global cancer statistics 2018: GLOBOCAN estimates of incidence and mortality worldwide for 36 cancers in

185 countries. CA Cancer J Clin 2018;68(6): 394–424.

3. Ang KK, Harris J, Wheeler R, et al. Human papillomavirus and survival of patients with oropharyngeal cancer. N Engl J Med 2010;363(1):24–35.

4. Lydiatt W, O'Sullivan B, Patel S, et al. Major changes in head and neck staging for 2018. Am Soc Clin Oncol Educ Book 2018;38:505–14.

5. Adelstein DJ, Saxton JP, Lavertu P, et al. A phase III randomized trial comparing concurrent chemotherapy and radiotherapy with radiotherapy alone in resectable stage III and IV squamous cell head and neck cancer: preliminary results. Head Neck 1997;19:567–75.

6. Brizel DM, Albers ME, Fisher SR, et al. Hyperfractionated irradiation with or without concurrent chemotherapy for locally advanced head and neck cancer. N Engl J Med 1998;338: 1798–804.

7. Peters LJ, Goepfert H, Ang KK, et al. Evaluation of the dose for postoperative radiation therapy of head and neck cancer: First report of a prospective randomized trial. Int J Radiat Oncol Biol Phys 1993; 26:3–11.

8. Bernier J, Cooper JS, Pajak TF, et al. Defining risk levels in locally advanced head and neck cancers: a comparative analysis of concurrent postoperative radiation plus chemotherapy trials of the EORTC (#22931) and RTOG (# 9501). Head Neck 2005; 27(10):843–50.

9. Heron DE, Ferris RL, Karamouzis M, et al. Stereotactic body radiotherapy for recurrent squamous cell carcinoma of the head and neck: results of a phase I dose-escalation trial. Int J Radiat Oncol Biol Phys 2009;75(5):1493–500.

10. Ling DC, Vargo JA, Ferris RL, et al. Risk of severe toxicity according to site of recurrence in patients treated with stereotactic body radiation therapy for recurrent head and neck cancer. Int J Radiat Oncol Biol Phys 2016;95(3):973–80.

11. Scott JG, Berglund A, Schell MJ, et al. A genome-based model for adjusting radiotherapy dose (GARD): a retrospective, cohort-based study. Lancet Oncol 2017;18(2):202–11.

12. Giraud P, Giraud P, Gasnier A, et al. Radiomics and machine learning for radiotherapy in head and neck cancers. Front Oncol 2019;9:174.

13. Wu J, Tha KK, Xing L, et al. Radiomics and radiogenomics for precision radiotherapy. J Radiat Res 2018;59(suppl_1):i25–31.

14. Kashani R, Olsen JR. Magnetic resonance imaging for target delineation and daily treatment modification. Semin Radiat Oncol 2018;28(3):178–84.

15. Heukelom J, Fuller CD. Head and neck cancer adaptive radiation therapy (ART): conceptual considerations for the informed clinician. Semin Radiat Oncol 2019;29(3):258–73.

16. Kabadi SJ, Fatterpekar GM, Anzai Y, et al. Dynamic contrast-enhanced MR imaging in head and neck cancer. Magn Reson Imaging Clin N Am 2018; 26(1):135–49.

17. Srinivasan A, Mohan S, Mukherji SK. Biologic imaging of head and neck cancer: the present and the future. AJNR Am J Neuroradiol 2012;33(4):586–94.

18. Vaupel P, Kallinowski F, Okunieff P. Blood flow, oxygen and nutrient supply, and metabolic microenvironment of human tumors: a review. Cancer Res 1989;49:6449–65.

19. Wong KH, Panek R, Bhide SA, et al. The emerging potential of magnetic resonance imaging in personalizing radiotherapy for head and neck cancer: an oncologist's perspective. Br J Radiol 2017; 90(1071):20160768.

20. Quon H, Brizel DM. Predictive and prognostic role of functional imaging of head and neck squamous cell carcinomas. Semin Radiat Oncol 2012;22(3): 220–32.

21. Davis AJ, Rehmani R, Srinivasan A, et al. Perfusion and permeability imaging for head and neck cancer: theory, acquisition, postprocessing, and relevance to clinical imaging. Magn Reson Imaging Clin N Am 2018;26(1):19–35.

22. Widmann G, Henninger B, Kremser C, et al. MRI sequences in head & neck radiology - State of the art. Rofo 2017;189(5):413–22.

23. Tofts PS, Kermode AG. Measurement of the blood-brain barrier permeability and leakage space using dynamic MR imaging. 1. Fundamental concepts. Magn Reson Med 1991;17:357–67.

24. Tofts PS, Brix G, Buckley DL, et al. Estimating kinetic parameters from dynamic\ contrast-enhanced T(1)-weighted MRI of a diffusable tracer: standardized quantities and symbols. J Magn Reson Imaging 1999;10:223–32.

25. Graff BA, Benjaminsen IC, Brurberg KG, et al. Comparison of tumorblood perfusion assessed by dynamic contrast-enhanced MRI with tumor blood supply assessed by invasive imaging. J Magn Reson Imaging 2005;21:272–81.

26. Newbold K, Partridge M, Cook G, et al. Advanced imaging applied to radiotherapy planning in head and neck cancer: a clinical review. Br J Radiol 2006;79(943):554–61.

27. Cooper RA, Carrington BM, Loncaster JA, et al. Tumour oxygenation levels correlate with dynamic contrast-enhanced magnetic resonance imaging parameters in carcinoma of the cervix. Radiother Oncol 2000;57:53–9.

28. Brizel DM, Sibley GS, Prosnitz LR, et al. Tumor hypoxia adversely effects the prognosis of carcinoma of the head and neck. Int J Radiat Oncol Biol Phys 1997;38(2):285–9.

29. Hermans R, Meijerink M, Van den Bogaert, et al. Tumor perfusion rate determined noninvasively by

dynamic computed tomography predicts outcome in head-and-neck cancer after radiotherapy. Int J Radiat Oncol Biol Phys 2003;57(5):1351–6.

30. Brown JM, Wilson WR. Exploiting tumour hypoxia in cancer treatment. Nat Rev Cancer 2004;4:437–47.

31. Newbold K, Castellano I, Charles-Edwards E, et al. An exploratory study into the role of dynamic contrast-enhanced magnetic resonance imaging or perfusion computed tomography for detection of intratumoral hypoxia in head-and-neck cancer. Int J Radiat Oncol Biol Phys 2009;74(1):29–37.

32. Donaldson SB, Betts G, Bonington SC, et al. Perfusion estimated with rapid dynamic contrast-enhanced magnetic resonance imaging correlates inversely with vascular endothelial growth factor expression and pimonidazole staining in head-and-neck cancer: a pilot study. Int J Radiat Oncol Biol Phys 2011;81(4):1176–83.

33. Jensen RL, Mumert ML, Gillespie DL, et al. Preoperative dynamic contrast-enhanced MRI correlates with molecular markers of hypoxia and vascularity in specific areas of intratumoral microenvironment and is predictive of patient outcome. Neuro Oncol 2014;16(2):280–91.

34. Hoskin PJ, Saunders MI, Goodchild K, et al. Dynamic contrast enhanced magnetic resonance scanning as a predictor of response to accelerated radiotherapy for advanced head and neck cancer. Br J Radiol 1999;72:1093–8.

35. Noij DP, de Jong MC, Mulders LG, et al. Contrast-enhanced perfusion magnetic resonance imaging for head and neck squamous cell carcinoma: a systematic review. Oral Oncol 2015;51(2):124–38.

36. Wang P, Popovtzer A, Eisbruch A, et al. An approach to identify, from DCE MRI, significant subvolumes of tumors related to outcomes in advanced head-and-neck cancer. Med Phys 2012;39(8):5277–85.

37. Aryal MP, Lee C, Hawkins PG, et al. Real-time quantitative assessment of accuracy and precision of blood volume derived from DCE-MRI in individual patients during a clinical trial. Tomography 2019;5(1):61–7.

38. Bhatnagar P, Subesunghe M, Patel C, et al. Functional imaging for radiation treatment planning, response assessment, and adaptive therapy in head and neck cancer. RadioGraphics 2013;33: 1909–29.

39. Castelli J, Simon A, Rigaud B, et al. Adaptive radiotherapy in head and neck cancer is required to avoid tumor underdose. Acta Oncol 2018;57(9): 1267–70.

40. Caudell JJ, Torres-Roca JF, Gillies RJ, et al. The future of personalised radiotherapy for head and neck cancer. Lancet Oncol 2017;18(5):e266–73.

41. El Beltagi, Elsotouhy AH, Own AM, et al. Functional magnetic resonance imaging of head and neck cancer: Performance and potential. Neuroradiol J 2019;32(1):36–52.

42. Elhalawani H, Ger RB, Mohamed ASR, et al. Joint head and neck radiotherapy-MRI development co-operative, Dynamic contrast-enhanced magnetic resonance imaging for head and neck cancers. Sci Data 2018;5:180008.

43. King AD, Chow SK, Yu KH, et al. DCE-MRI for pretreatment prediction and post-treatment assessment of treatment response in sites of squamous cell carcinoma in the head and neck. PLoS One 2015;10(12):e0144770.

44. Margalit DN, Schoenfeld JD, Tishler RB, et al. Radiation oncology–new approaches in squamous cell cancer of the head and neck. Hematol Oncol Clin North Am 2015;29(6):1093–106.

45. Metcalfe P, Liney GP, Holloway L, et al. The potential for an enhanced role for MRI in radiation-therapy treatment planning. Technol Cancer Res Treat 2013;12(5):429–46.

46. Wan DQ. Advances in functional imaging in the assessment of head and neck cancer. Oral Maxillofac Surg Clin North Am 2019;31(4):627–35.

47. You D, Aryal M, Samuels SE, et al. Temporal feature extraction from DCE-MRI to identify poorly perfused subvolumes of tumors related to outcomes of radiation therapy in head and neck cancer. Tomography 2016;2(4):341–52.

48. Press RH, Shu HG, Shim H, et al. The use of quantitative imaging in radiation oncology: a Quantitative Imaging Network (QIN) Perspective. Int J Radiat Oncol Biol Phys 2018;102(4):1219–35.

49. Bammer R. Basic principles of diffusion-weighted imaging. Eur J Radiol 2003;45:169–84.

50. Le Bihan D. Apparent diffusion coefficient and beyond: what diffusion MR imaging can tell us about tissue structure. Radiology 2013;268: 318–22.

51. Yun TJ, Kim JH, Kim KH, et al. Head and neck squamous cell carcinoma: differentiation of histologic grade with standard- and high-b-value diffusion-weighted MRI. Head Neck 2013;35:626–31.

52. Wang J, Takashima S, Takayama F, et al. Head and neck lesions: characterization with diffusion-weighted echo-planar MR imaging. Radiology 2001;220:621–30.

53. Driessen JP, Caldas-Magalhaes J, Janssen LM, et al. Diffusion-weighted MR imaging in laryngeal and hypopharyngeal carcinoma: association between apparent diffusion coefficient and histologic findings. Radiology 2014;272:456–63.

54. de Bondt RB, Hoeberigs MC, Nelemans PJ, et al. Diagnostic accuracy and additional value of diffusion-weighted imaging for discrimination of malignant cervical lymph nodes in head and neck squamous cell carcinoma. Neuroradiology 2009; 51:183–92.

55. Vandecaveye V, De Keyzer F, Vander Poorten V, et al. Head and neck squamous cell carcinoma: value of diffusion-weighted MR imaging for nodal staging. Radiology 2009;251:134–46.

56. Srinivasan A, Dvorak R, Perni K, et al. Differentiation of benign and malignant pathology in the head and neck using 3T apparent diffusion coefficient values: early experience. AJNR Am J Neuroradiol 2008;29:40–4.

57. Sakamoto J, Yoshino N, Okochi K, et al. Tissue characterization of head and neck lesions using diffusion-weighted MR imaging with SPLICE. Eur J Radiol 2009;69:260–8.

58. Chernock RD, El-Mofty SK, Thorstad WL, et al. HPV-related nonkeratinizing squamous cell carcinoma of the oropharynx: utility of microscopic features in predicting patient outcome. Head Neck Pathol 2009;3:186–94.

59. de Perrot T, Lenoir V, Domingo Ayllon M, et al. Apparent diffusion coefficient histograms of human papillomavirus-positive and human papillomavirus-negative head and neck squamous cell carcinoma: assessment of tumor heterogeneity and comparison with histopathology. AJNR Am J Neuroradiol 2017;38:2153–60.

60. King AD, Thoeny HC. Functional MRI for the prediction of treatment response in head and neck squamous cell carcinoma: potential and limitations. Cancer Imaging 2016;16:23.

61. Kim S, Loevner L, Quon H, et al. Diffusion-weighted magnetic resonance imaging for predicting and detecting early response to chemoradiation therapy of squamous cell carcinomas of the head and neck. Clin Cancer Res 2009;15:986–94.

62. Nakajo M, Nakajo M, Kajiya Y, et al. FDG PET/CT and diffusion-weighted imaging of head and neck squamous cell carcinoma: comparison of prognostic significance between primary tumor standardized uptake value and apparent diffusion coefficient. Clin Nucl Med 2012;37:475–80.

63. Matoba M, Tuji H, Shimode Y, et al. Fractional change in apparent diffusion coefficient as an imaging biomarker for predicting treatment response in head and neck cancer treated with chemoradiotherapy. AJNR Am J Neuroradiol 2014;35:379–85.

64. Vandecaveye V, Dirix P, De Keyzer F, et al. Diffusion-weighted magnetic resonance imaging early after chemoradiotherapy to monitor treatment response in head-and-neck squamous cell carcinoma. Int J Radiat Oncol Biol Phys 2012;82:1098–107.

65. King AD, Mo FK, Yu KH, et al. Squamous cell carcinoma of the head and neck: diffusion-weighted MR imaging for prediction and monitoring of treatment response. Eur Radiol 2010;20:2213–20.

66. Abdel Razek AA, Kandeel AY, et al. Role of diffusion-weighted echo-planar MR imaging in differentiation of residual or recurrent head and neck tumors and posttreatment changes. AJNR Am J Neuroradiol 2007;28:1146–52.

67. Vandecaveye V, De Keyzer F, Nuyts S, et al. Detection of head and neck squamous cell carcinoma with diffusion weighted MRI after (chemo)radiotherapy: correlation between radiologic and histopathologic findings. Int J Radiat Oncol Biol Phys 2007;67:960–71.

68. Driessen JP, van Kempen PM, van der Heijden GJ, et al. Diffusion-weightedimaging in head and neck squamous cell carcinomas: a systematic review. Head Neck 2015;37:440–8.

69. Payabvash S. Quantitative diffusion magnetic resonance imaging in head and neck tumors. Quant Imaging Med Surg 2018;8(10):1052–65.

70. Fujima N, Sakashita T, Homma A, et al. Advanced diffusion models in head and neck squamous cell carcinoma patients: Goodness of fit, relationships among diffusion parameters and comparison with dynamic contrast-enhanced perfusion. Magn Reson Imaging 2017;36:16–23.

71. Fujima N, Yoshida D, Sakashita T, et al. Intravoxel incoherent motion diffusion-weighted imaging in head and neck squamous cell carcinoma: assessment of perfusion-related parameters compared to dynamic contrast enhanced MRI. Magn Reson Imaging 2014;32:1206–13.

72. Fujima N, Kudo K, Yoshida D, et al. Arterial spinlabeling to determine tumor viability in head and neck cancer before and after treatment. J Magn Reson Imaging 2014;40(4):920–8.

73. Chen Y, Ren W, Zheng D, et al. Diffusion kurtosis imaging predicts neoadjuvant chemotherapy responses within 4 days in advanced nasopharyngeal carcinoma patients. J Magn Reson Imaging 2015;42:1354–61.

74. Chen WB, Zhang B, Liang L, et al. To predict the radiosensitivity of nasopharyngeal carcinoma using intravoxel incoherent motion MRI at 3.0 T. Oncotarget 2017;8(32):53740–50.

75. Galban CJ, Mukherji SK, Chenevert TL, et al. A feasibility study of parametric response map analysis of diffusion-weighted magnetic resonance imaging scans of head and neck cancer patients for providing early detection of therapeutic efficacy. Transl Oncol 2009;2(3):184–90.

76. Rijpkema M, Kaanders J, Joosten F, et al. Effects of breathing a hyperoxic hypercapnic gas mixture on blood oxygenation and vascularity of head and neck tumors as measured by magnetic resonance imaging. Int J Radiat Oncol Biol Phys Med Biol 2002;53:1185–91.

77. Kotas M, Schmitt P, Jakob PM, et al. Monitoring of tumor oxygenation changes in head-and-neck carcinoma patients breathing a hyperoxic hypercapnic gas mixture with a noninvasive

MRI technique. Strahlenther Onkol 2009;185:
19–26.

78. Li XS, Fan HX, Fang H, et al. Value of R2* obtained from T2*-weighted imaging in predicting the prognosis of advanced cervical squamous carcinoma treated with concurrent chemoradiotherapy. J Magn Reson Imaging 2015;42:681–8.

79. Abdel Razek AA, Poptani H. MR spectroscopy of head and neck cancer. Eur J Radiol 2013;82(6): 982–9.

80. Differding S, Hanin FX, Gregoire V. PET imaging biomarkers in head and neck cancer. Eur J Nucl Med Mol Imaging 2015;42(4):613–22.

81. Jansen JF, Schöder H, Lee NY, et al. Tumor metabolism and perfusion in head and neck squamous cell carcinoma: pretreatment multimodality imaging with (1)H magnetic resonance spectroscopy, dynamic contrast-enhanced MRI, and [(18)F]FDG-PET. Int J Radiat Oncol Biol Phys 2012;82:299–307.

82. Rana L, Sharma S, Sood S, et al. Volumetric CT perfusion assessment of treatment response in head and neck squamous cell carcinoma: comparison of CT perfusion parameters before and after chemoradiation therapy. Eur J Radiol Open 2015; 2:46–54.

83. Forghani R, De Man B, Gupta R. Dual-energy computed tomography: physical principles, approaches to scanning, usage, and implementation: part 2. Neuroimaging Clin N Am 2017;27(3): 385–400.

84. Forghani R, De Man B, Gupta R. Dual-energy computed tomography: physical principles, approaches to scanning, usage, and implementation: part 1. Neuroimaging Clin N Am 2017;27(3): 371–84.

85. Forghani R, Srinivasan A, Forghani B. Advanced tissue characterization and texture analysis using dual-energy computed tomography: Horizons and emerging applications. Neuroimaging Clin N Am 2017;27(3):533–46.

86. McCollough CH, Leng S, Yu L, et al. Dual- and multi-energy CT: principles, technical approaches, and clinical applications. Radiology 2015;276(3): 637–53.

87. Albrecht MH, Scholtz JE, Kraft J, et al. Assessment of an advanced monoenergetic reconstruction technique in dual-energy computed tomography of head and neck cancer. Eur Radiol 2015;25(8): 2493–501.

88. Forghani R. An update on advanced dual-energy CT for head and neck cancer imaging. Expert Rev Anticancer Ther 2019;19(7):633–44.

89. Forghani R, Kelly H, Yu E, et al. Low-energy virtual monochromatic dual-energy computed tomography images for the evaluation of head and neck squamous cell carcinoma: a study of tumor visibility compared with single-energy computed

tomography and user acceptance. J Comput Assist Tomogr 2017;41(4):565–71.

90. Forghani R, Kelly HR, Curtin HD. Applications of dual-energy computed tomography for the evaluation of head and neck squamous cell carcinoma. Neuroimaging Clin N Am 2017;27(3):445–59.

91. Kraft M, Ibrahim M, Spector M, et al. Comparison of virtual monochromatic series, iodine overlay maps, and single energy CT equivalent images in head and neck cancer conspicuity. Clin Imaging 2018; 48:26–31.

92. Wichmann JL, Nöske EM, Kraft J, et al. Virtual monoenergetic dual-energy computed tomography: optimization of kiloelectron volt settings in head and neck cancer. Invest Radiol 2014;49(11): 735–41.

93. Lam S, Gupta R, Levental M, et al. Optimal virtual monochromatic images for evaluation of normal tissues and head and neck cancer using dual-energy CT. AJNR Am J Neuroradiol 2015;36(8): 1518–24.

94. Perez-Lara A, Forghani R. Dual-energy computed tomography of the neck: a pictorial review of normal anatomy, variants, and pathologic entities using different energy reconstructions and material decomposition maps. Neuroimaging Clin N Am 2017;27(3):499–522.

95. Srinivasan A, Parker RA, Manjunathan A, et al. Differentiation of benign and malignant neck pathologies: preliminary experience using spectral computed tomography. J Comput Assist Tomogr 2013;37(5):666–72.

96. Yamauchi H, Buehler M, Goodsitt MM, et al. Dual-energy CT-based differentiation of benign post-treatment changes from primary or recurrent malignancy of the head and neck: comparison of spectral hounsfield units at 40 and 70 keV and iodine concentration. AJR Am J Roentgenol 2016; 206(3):580–7.

97. Forghani R, Levental M, Gupta R, et al. Different spectral hounsfield unit curve and high-energy virtual monochromatic image characteristics of squamous cell carcinoma compared with nonossified thyroid cartilage. AJNR Am J Neuroradiol 2015; 36(6):1194–200.

98. Kuno H, Sakamaki K, Fujii S, et al. Comparison of MR imaging and dual-energy CT for the evaluation of cartilage invasion by laryngeal and hypopharyngeal squamous cell carcinoma. AJNR Am J Neuroradiol 2018;39(3):524–31.

99. Kuno H, Onaya H, Iwata R, et al. Evaluation of cartilage invasion by laryngeal and hypopharyngeal squamous cell carcinoma with dual-energy CT. Radiology 2012;265(2):488–96.

100. Bahig H, Lapointe A, Bedwani S, et al. Dual-energy computed tomography for prediction of locoregional recurrence after radiotherapy in larynx

and hypopharynx squamous cell carcinoma. Eur J Radiol 2019;110:1–6.

101. Nair JR, DeBlois F, Ong T, et al. Dual-energy CT: 2er. J Comput Assist Tomogr 2017;41(6):931–6.

102. Hudobivnik N, Schwarz F, Johnson T, et al. Comparison of proton therapy treatment planning for head tumors with a pencil beam algorithm on dual and single energy CT images. Am Assoc Phys Med 2016;43:495–504.

103. Kastrinidis N, Kuhn FP, Hany TF, et al. 18F-FDG-PET/CT for the assessment of the contralateral neck in patients with head and neck squamous cell carcinoma. Laryngoscope 2013;123(5): 1210–5.

104. Troost EG, Schinagl DA, Bussink J, et al. Innovations in radiotherapy planning of head and neck cancers: role of PET. J Nucl Med 2010;51:66–76.

105. Kresnik E, Mikosch P, Gallowitsch HJ, et al. Evaluation of head and neck cancer with 18F-FDG PET: a comparison with conventional methods. Eur J Nucl Med 2001;28:816–21.

106. Riegel AC, Berson AM, Destian S, et al. Variability of gross tumor volume delineation in head-and-neck cancer using CT and PET/CT fusion. Int J Radiat Oncol Biol Phys 2006;65(3):726–32.

107. Paulino AC, Koshy M, Howell R, et al. Comparison of CT- and FDG-PET-defined gross tumor volume in intensity-modulated radiotherapy for head-and-neck cancer. Int J Radiat Oncol Biol Phys 2005; 61(5):1385–92.

108. Geets X, Tomsej M, Lee JA, et al. Adaptive biological image-guided IMRT with anatomic and functional imaging in pharyngo-laryngeal tumors: impact on target volume delineation and dose distribution using helical tomotherapy. Radiother Oncol 2007;85(1):105–15.

109. Castadot P, Geets X, Lee JA, et al. Assessment by a deformable registration method of the volumetric and positional changes of target volumes and organs at risk in pharyngo-laryngeal tumors treated with concomitant chemo-radiation. Radiother Oncol 2010;95(2):209–17.

110. Bentzen SM, Gregoire V. Molecular imaging-based dose painting: a novel paradigm for radiation therapy prescription. Semin Radiat Oncol 2011;21(2): 101–10.

111. Madani I, Duprez F, Boterberg T, et al. Maximum tolerated dose in a phase I trial on adaptive dose painting by numbers for head and neck cancer. Radiother Oncol 2011;101(3):351–5.

112. Ling CC, Larson S, Amols H, et al. Towards multidimensional radiotherapy (MD-CRT): biological imaging and biological conformality. Int J Radiat Oncol Biol Phys 2000;47(3):551–60.

113. Dirix P, Vandecaveye V, De Keyzer F, et al. Dose painting in radiotherapy for head and neck squamous cell carcinoma: value of repeated functional imaging with (18)F-FDG PET, (18)F-fluoromisonidazole PET, diffusion-weighted MRI, and dynamic contrast-enhanced MRI. J Nucl Med 2009;50(7): 1020–7.

114. Koukourakis MI, Bentzen SM, Giatromanolaki A, et al. Endogenous markers of two separate hypoxiaresponse pathways (hypoxia inducible factor 2 alpha and carbonicanhydrase 9) are associated with radiotherapy failure in head and neck cancer patients recruited in the CHART randomized trial. J Clin Oncol 2006;24(5):727–35.

115. Tamaki N, Hirata K. Tumor hypoxia: a new PET imaging biomarker in clinical oncology. Int J Clin Oncol 2016;21(4):619–25.

116. Okamoto S, Shiga T, Yasuda K, et al. High reproducibility of tumor hypoxia evaluated by 18F-fluoromisonidazole PET for head and neck cancer. J Nucl Med 2013;54(2):201–7.

117. Verma V, Choi JI, Sawant A, et al. Use of PET and other functional imaging to guide target delineation in radiation oncology. Semin Radiat Oncol 2018; 28(3):171–7.

118. Hoeben BA, Bussink J, Troost EG, et al. Molecular PET imaging for biology-guided adaptive radiotherapy of head and neck cancer. Acta Oncol 2013;52(7):1257–71.

119. Thorwarth D, Eschmann SM, Paulsen F, et al. Hypoxia dose painting by numbers: a planning study. Int J Radiat Oncol Biol Phys 2007;68(1):291–300.

120. Weber WA. Monitoring tumor response to therapy with 18F-FLT PET. J Nucl Med 2010;51(6):841–4.

121. Shields AF, Grierson JR, Dohmen BM, et al. Imaging proliferation in vivo with [F-18]FLT and positron emission tomography. Nat Med 1998;4:1334–6.

122. Cobben DC, van der Laan BF, Maas B, et al. 8F-FLT PET for visualization of laryngeal cancer: comparison with 18F-FDG PET. J Nucl Med 2004;45: 226–31.

123. Hoeben BA, Troost EG, Span PN, et al. 18F-FLT PET during radiotherapy or chemoradiotherapy in head and neck squamous cell carcinoma is an early predictor of outcome. J Nucl Med 2013;54: 532–40.

124. Troost EG, Bussink J, Hoffmann AL, et al. 18F-FLT PET/CT for early response monitoring and dose escalation in oropharyngeal tumors. J Nucl Med 2010;51(6):866–74.

125. Al-Ibraheem A, Buck A, Krause BJ, et al. Clinical applications of FDG PET and PET/CT in head and neck cancer. J Oncol 2009;2009:1–13.

126. Beer AJ, Haubner R, Sarbia M, et al. Positron emission tomography using [18F]Galacto-RGD identifies the level of integrin alpha(v)beta3 expression in man. Clin Cancer Res 2006;12(13): 3942–9.

127. Haubner R, Weber WA, Beer AJ, et al. Noninvasive visualization of the activated alphavbeta3 integrin

in cancer patients by positron emission tomography and [18F]galacto-RGD. PLoS Med 2005;2(3): 244–52.

128. Schoder H, Fury M, Lee N, et al. PET monitoring of therapy response in head and neck squamous cell carcinoma. J Nucl Med 2009;50(suppl 1):74S–88S.

129. Chen SH, Wang HM, Lin CY, et al. RGD-K5 PET/CT in patients with advanced head and neck cancer treated with concurrent chemoradiotherapy: results from a pilot study. Eur J Nucl Med Mol Imaging 2016;43(9):1621–9.

130. Li W, Niu G, Lang L, et al. PET imaging of EGF receptors using [18F]FBEM-EGF in a head and neck squamous cell carcinoma model. Eur J Nucl Med Mol Imaging 2012;39(2):300–8.

131. Mena E, Thippsandra S, Yanamadala A, et al. Molecular imaging and precision medicine in head and neck cancer. PET Clin 2017;12(1):7–25.

132. Huizing FJ, Garousi J, Lok J, et al. CAIX-targeting radiotracers for hypoxia imaging in head and neck cancer models. Sci Rep 2019;9(1):18898.

133. Huizing FJ, Hoeben BAW, Franssen G, et al. Quantitative imaging of the hypoxia-related marker CAIX in head and neck squamous cell carcinoma xenograft models. Mol Pharm 2019;16(2):701–8.

134. Lambin P, Rios-Velazquez E, Leijenaar R, et al. Radiomics: extracting more information from medical images using advanced feature analysis. Eur J Cancer 2012;48(4):441–6.

135. Kumar V, Gu Y, Basu S, et al. Radiomics: the process and the challenges. Magn Reson Imaging 2012;30(9):1234–48.

136. Gillies RJ, Kinahan PE, Hricak H. Radiomics: images are more than pictures, they are data. Radiology 2016;278(2):563–77.

137. Forghani R, Savadjiev P, Chatterjee A, et al. Radiomics and artificial intelligence for biomarker and prediction model development in oncology. Comput Struct Biotechnol J 2019;12(17):995–1008.

138. Seidler M, Forghani B, Reinhold C, et al. Dual-energy CT texture analysis with machine learning for the evaluation and characterization of cervical lymphadenopathy. Comput Struct Biotechnol J 2019;16(17):1009–15.

139. Savadjiev P, Chong J, Dohan A, et al. Image-based biomarkers for solid tumor quantification. Eur Radiol 2019;29(10):5431–40.

140. Al Ajmi E, Forghani B, et al. Spectral multi-energy CT texture analysis with machine learning for tissue classification: an investigation using classification of benign parotid tumours as a testing paradigm. Eur Radiol 2018;28(6):2604–11.

141. Forghani R, Chatterjee A, Reinhold C, et al. Head and neck squamous cell carcinoma: prediction of cervical lymph node metastasis by dual-energy CT texture analysis with machine learning. Eur Radiol 2019;29(11):6172–81.

Artificial Intelligence in Head and Neck Imaging
A Glimpse into the Future

Kyle Werth, MD[a], Luke Ledbetter, MD[b],*

KEYWORDS

• Artificial intelligence • Machine learning • Deep learning • Automation • Head and neck imaging

KEY POINTS

- Artificial intelligence (AI) in imaging can improve efficiency, quality, and automation of tasks frequently encountered in radiology practices.
- Technical and statistical details in AI are complex, but familiarity of common terms and broad concepts is important for radiologists as AI becomes more commonplace.
- Machine learning and deep learning models can improve patient care throughout clinical workflow from the time of imaging, to interpretation, and through to quality improvement.
- Head and neck imaging is prime for AI integration due to the challenge of image acquisition and interpretation together with abundant clinical and pathologic correlative data.
- AI faces numerous internal and external challenges to widespread clinical adoption.

INTRODUCTION

Throughout human history, individuals have sought ways to make processes more efficient and effective through invention and industrialization. Over the past 20 years, improved imaging techniques, digitization, and methods to move, store, and display imaging information have resulted in massive improvements in the efficiency and effectiveness of radiologists. Radiology was at the forefront of the digitization of medicine. Now with the massive amount of imaging data and improved computational power of computer processors, the next step in improved efficiency and effectiveness is on the doorstep of radiology practice—artificial intelligence (AI).

The term AI was coined at a conference at Dartmouth College in 1956, where the field of AI research was first established.[1] The definition of AI varies slightly from source to source, with the overarching core concept of a machine mimicking human cognitive functions. Throughout the remainder of the twentieth century, interest in the discipline of AI ebbed and flowed but remained largely hypothetical. Over the past ten years, the application of AI to the field of medicine garnered much more attention. This renewed focus on AI was the direct result of the massive amounts of digital information, known as big data, produced during the information age.[1] Computer processing power simultaneously improved, and rapid processing of large amounts of data became feasible and commonplace. Together, the large amount of digital data and computer processing advances allowed computation-heavy AI models to be possible. Given radiology's early digitization and the ability to store and organize data, radiology is uniquely positioned to be a leader in the next era, incorporating AI into the field of medicine.[1]

This article defines and briefly describes common technical concepts in AI, such as machine and deep learning. After the background of

a Department of Radiology, University of Kansas Medical Center, 3901 Rainbow Boulevard, Mailstop 4032, Kansas City, KS 66160, USA; b Department of Radiology, David Geffen School of Medicine at UCLA, 757 Westwood Plaza, Suite 1621D, Los Angeles, CA 90095, USA
* Corresponding author.
E-mail address: lledbetter@mednet.ucla.edu
Twitter: @LNLedbetter (L.L.)

Neuroimag Clin N Am 30 (2020) 359–368
https://doi.org/10.1016/j.nic.2020.04.004
1052-5149/20/© 2020 Elsevier Inc. All rights reserved.

techniques is described, current and potential applications in general radiology as well as head and neck imaging are covered. Finally, current challenges and barriers to the application of AI techniques into clinical practice are discussed.

MACHINE AND DEEP LEARNING

This section briefly describes basic technical concepts used in radiology-based AI. AI applications in head and neck imaging largely are early in development, with integration into the clinical environment in a nascent stage. Widespread adoption and integration of AI into clinical workflows, however, are not far in the future. Basic understanding of terms and concepts allows for better comprehension of the medical literature, collaboration with data scientists, and participation in the decision-making processes required before workflow integration. A short list of key terms and definitions discussed in the section is included in **Table 1**. The following sections are designed to be an introduction to terms and concepts frequently encountered in radiology AI applications and not a comprehensive review.

Machine Learning

Machine learning is the subset of AI used most broadly in radiology[2] (**Fig. 1**). The term, *learning*, differs from *programming* in computers. A program is detailed instructions to get from an input to a desired output. Learning, on the other hand, tackles situations where there is no obvious program. The input is known, but the best steps to get from input to output are unknown. Machine learning uses framework architecture to evaluate the input data using self-modifying variables. The modifiable variables are referred to as weights. The model continues altering weights repetitively until the output closely matches the desired result. When no further improvement can be made, it can be said the model has learned how to arrive at the desired output. For example, an input can be a T2 image of the face and the desired output is segmenting the parotid glands from all other tissues in the face. The algorithm processes the image by extracting detailed digital information, manipulating the extracted information to attempt to classify the original image data as normal parotid tissue versus not parotid tissue, and then comparing the results to the examples prelabeled with the desired outcome, also known as the ground truth. The program repeats the process, each time slightly changing the calculations to optimize the results, until no further improvements can be made. It can then be

Table 1	
Common terms encountered in imaging artificial intelligence	
Artificial intelligence	Machine activity mimicking human cognitive functions, such as learning or problem solving
Machine learning	Computer algorithm producing predictions without explicit instructions on how to arrive at the final prediction
Feature	Measurable characteristic of imaging data
Node	Computational unit receiving 1 or more inputs, applies function to inputs, and gives output based on an activation threshold
Layer	Collection of nodes at a specific depth of the network
Weight	Modifiable variable to define strength of connection between nodes and layers
Neural networks	Machine learning architecture modeled after the structure and function of biologic neural systems consisting of nodes, layers, and connections
Deep learning	Neural network architecture with an increased number of layers
Convoluted neural network	Type of deep neural network, inspired by the visual cortex, with fewer required parameters and more tolerant to image irregularities (rotation, translation, etc.)
Natural language processing	Computer interaction with and extraction of data from written or spoken language

said that the computer learned to segment the parotid glands. In addition, the machine learning model potentially can adapt and improve the output results with continued input of imaging data after the model is validated.

Machine Learning Methods

Machine learning algorithms can learn by supervised, unsupervised, or reinforcement methods. Supervised learning, as described in the parotid

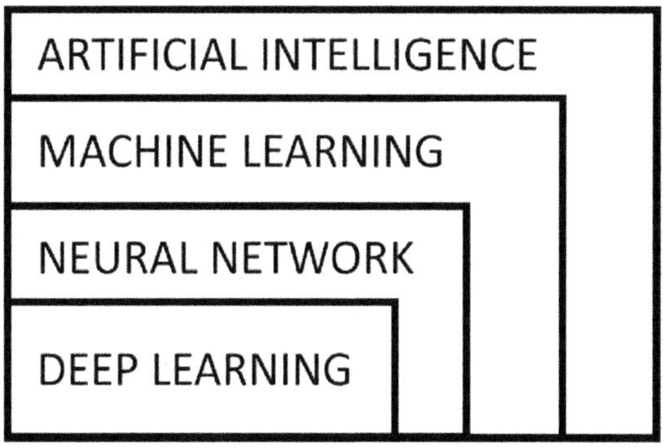

Fig. 1. Hierarchy of AI common in radiology.

gland segmentation example, discussed previously, is when the model is trained with ground truth–labeled examples. Supervised machine learning techniques are some of the most frequently encountered and relevant AI techniques in radiology.[3] Unsupervised learning models evaluate the input data without the desired ground truth defined. The unsupervised learning algorithm attempts to find relationships within the data and divides the results into similar groups based on its processing, not based on ground truth training examples. Examples of supervised and unsupervised machine learning techniques are listed in Box 1 and can be used as a reference when reading about machine learning applications. Lastly, reinforcement machine learning models use concepts of both supervised and unsupervised models. The model initially is built using labeled data, like supervised learning, but continues to improve classifications using unlabeled data, similar to unsupervised learning.

Neural Networks

One of the more common machine learning architectures is a neural network. Neural networks are modeled after biologic neural systems and consist of multiple nodes (analogous to neurons) arranged in layers with extensive interconnectivity between layers (axons). The layers are arranged by input and output layers with 1 or more hidden layer(s) of nodes in-between. The nodes are connected to all other nodes in the preceding and following layers. Before an input value reaches a node, it is multiplied by a weight. Each node then applies a unique function to the weighted input value. If the resulting value meets an activation threshold, information is passed to all nodes in next layer (Fig. 2). Therefore, changing the weight values can increase or decrease the importance of a feature to the next node. The program essentially can alter the

weights of complex statistical data to produce different results similar to a person weighing evidence to come to a final conclusion based on the strengths and weakness of the presenting evidence.

Deep Learning and Convoluted Neural Networks

Deep learning is a further subset of machine learning and neural networks (Fig. 3). Deep learning refers to use of numerous, usually hidden, layers within the neural network, frequently more than 20 layers.[4] The increase in layers allows for a higher number and more complex features to be extracted from images. Deep learning models require a high level of computational power and only became viable in the previous decade due to advancements in graphics processing units used commonly for computer gaming.

Although learning models can extract numerous and complex features from images, imaging data of biologic processes often are heterogenous from data set to data set. Orientation of images, slice selection, motion, rotation, and variation of biologic sizes and shapes result in challenges for standard feature extractions. Convoluted neural networks are more robust in handling variations compared with other neural networks. The input data to each layer are passed through filters, called convolutions, which reduce parameters needed for feature detection. This allows more efficient processing and extraction of imaging features, such as edges and corners. As layers become down-sampled through convolutions, the network becomes more robust at identifying features in the presence of image variations.[5] Convoluted neural networks dominate computer vision techniques due to their power to handle variations in images. Simpler machine learning techniques may be more powerful, however, when data are more homogeneous and standardized. No single model is best for all tasks, and identification of the best model to perform desired tasks is necessary for optimal results.

ARTIFICIAL INTELLIGENCE IN GENERAL IMAGING AND HEAD AND NECK IMAGING
General Imaging

Hyperbole is common with new and emerging technologies and AI is no different. A perspective piece in The New England Journal of Medicine, published in 2016, suggested radiologists and anatomic pathologists would be replaced by AI in as little as 5 years.[6] Other prominent individuals, including University of Oxford economists, the founder of Google Brain deep learning

---

Box 1
Examples of common machine learning techniques classified by learning method

Supervised learning

- Support vector machine
- Decision tree
- Linear regression
- Logistic regression
- Naive Bayes classifier
- k-nearest neighbor
- Random forest
- Neural networks

Unsupervised learning

- k-means clustering
- Mean shift
- Affinity propagation
- Hierarchical clustering
- Gaussian mixture modeling
- Markov random fields

---

project, and AI luminaries outside of the field of radiology echoed similar opinions regarding the future domination of AI in radiology.[7–9] After the initial wave of hype around AI and radiology, expectations now have tempered.[10] Current focus now is on how AI can improve patient care through automation and efficiency as well as augmenting, not replacing, the current roles of the physician. AI will not solve all imaging problems but will be a powerful tool to improve the delivery of quality health care. Broad clinical concepts within radiology where AI currently is being applied are described and specific examples of AI application to head and neck imaging subsequently discussed.

Image acquisition

Machine learning and deep learning can be applied to the initial acquisition and processing of images. Automating this process can lead to shorter imaging times and improved diagnostic quality utilizing fewer data.[11] MR imaging as a modality is a prime candidate for this application because resolution often is associated with longer acquisition times, which limits the modality in emergency situations.[12] Faster acquisition times can be achieved by under-sampling k-space and reducing the data set used to create images. Traditional image reconstruction techniques produce lower-quality images with under-sampling of k-space. New deep learning techniques for reconstruction of k-space can estimate and fill in the under-sampled data, resulting in reduced imaging times while maintaining diagnostic-quality image reconstruction.[13–15] Similar to prolonged imaging times for MR imaging, computed tomography (CT) quality is related to radiation dose. Noise and artifacts reduce image quality in CT images acquired at lower radiation doses. AI algorithms can remove or reduce artifacts found with lower CT doses, such as streak artifact[16] or noise.[17] These techniques can allow low-dose CT to result in better resolution imaging with fewer artifacts. Intravascular contrast volume also can be decreased by utilizing deep learning techniques to create diagnostic-quality postcontrast MR images from under-dosed and low-dosed source images.[18]

Postprocessing

The ongoing development of high-resolution, complex imaging results in increasing clinical volume and complexity of images to be evaluated by a radiologist. Machine learning applications can assist with extraction of information from the examination prior to radiologist interpretation. A common first step in processing clinically relevant information from source data is tissue segmentation. Classic methods of segmentation require human expertise to identify the desired structures correctly and time to manually contour the edges or boundaries of the structures. Machine learning is adept at detecting important characteristics of objects within an image to divide 1 tissue or structure from an adjacent dissimilar structure. After accurate segmentation of a desired structure, automatic quantification of dimensions, volumes, texture characteristics, or changes from prior examinations can be determined immediately.[19–21] This information can be provided automatically to the interpreting radiologist and aid in efficiency and quality of interpretation.

Autodetection of findings

Applying similar segmentation techniques, described previously, abnormalities on an image can be detected from the adjacent normal or expected tissues. Computer-aided detection was introduced into radiology in the 1990s to much initial fanfare and did not live up the hype or potential after introduction into clinical workflows. Current versions of computer-aided detection utilizing deep learning models, however, commonly surpass human performance at simple detection tasks.[22] Computer-automated detection can be applied to images in several ways. One method is to risk-stratify imaging examinations prior to human evaluation. When applied to critical findings,

NODE

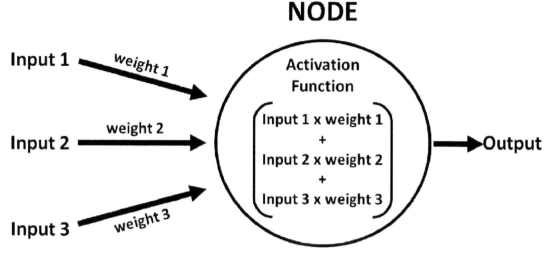

Fig. 2. Example of neural network node. Each input value represents a piece of information extracted from the source data, which is multiplied by a modifiable weight value. At the node, the values of the weighted inputs are totaled. The totaled value passes through an activation function and the result is passed to the next layer.

such as the detection of intracranial hemorrhage, the examination can be flagged automatically for urgent radiologist review on the worklist.[23] Computer-aided detection also can operate as an assistive tool for radiologists at the time of interpretation by detecting clinically important findings and providing automatic extraction of useful data from the lesion.

Image quality

Currently, most imaging practices place the responsibility of initial image quality control with the technician performing the examination. This subjective evaluation of quality can lead to patient recall and repeat imaging if the interpreting radiologist disagrees with the technologist's initial review. Deep learning tools can evaluate and score the quality of images prior to human evaluation, preventing time-consuming and expensive patient callbacks through immediate technologist feedback of quality.[24] Sources of imaging artifacts, such as patient movement, can be detected, quantified, and potentially corrected through deep learning processes.[25,26] Additional artifacts, such as metal artifact, cross-talk noise, and magnetic field inhomogeneity, also can be reduced through AI techniques.[12] Intelligent applications also can improve standardization of imaging by automatically detecting and selecting anatomic landmarks used to set the area of coverage for cross-sectional imaging examinations.

Reporting

Moving beyond image data, radiology reports contain a large volume of high-level information about images and cognitive summation of findings in impressions. Traditionally, extraction of data from narrative reports was time consuming and required an in-depth familiarity with the written language. Natural language processing is a type of machine learning that takes inputs in the form of narrative text, converts the text into structured data, and identifies and extracts information. Natural language processing has been used in disease surveillance by automated extraction of clinical important from multiple reports.[27] Natural language processing also has been applied to automated extraction and tracking of follow-up imaging recommendations within reports.[28]

Imaging integration with outside data

As discussed previously, AI's immediate impact likely will be augmentation to the daily practices of the radiologists. Radiologists usually do not interpret images in a vacuum. Additional information outside of the images are used to put every patient and image in context. This information frequently is obtained from imaging requests, patient care notes, laboratory or pathology reports, references, and the local public health environment. Automated integration of relevant patient or disease data from sources outside the imaging environment could augment the overall quality and efficiency of radiologists' practice. Heterogenous data and proprietary commercial data structures result in significant challenges for integration of data across platforms.[2,29]

Artificial Intelligence Applications in Head and Neck Imaging

Extensive work on AI application to head and neck imaging is well under way. Most current work is

INPUT LAYER   HIDDEN LAYERS   OUTPUT LAYER

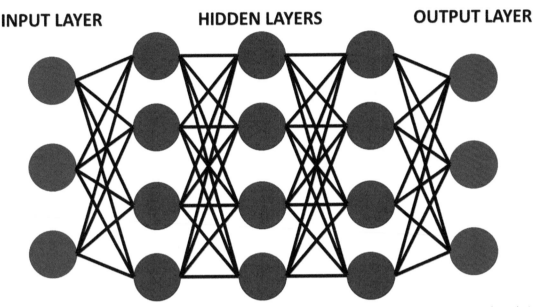

Fig. 3. Graphic representation of a deep neural network. Each node in a layer passes its output to each node in the next layer. Deep neural networks frequently contain multiple hidden layers between the model's input and output layers.

early in development and not yet integrated into widespread practice, but this review highlights several examples of emerging applications of AI in the field of head and neck imaging. The following described applications are only a brief glimpse to the work being done in AI in head and neck imaging. Future applications of AI to head and neck imaging described in this section builds on the several of the general concepts described previously.

Segmentation in the head and neck
As previously described, segmentation processes are important in identifying borders between an area of interest and its dissimilar neighboring areas. Segmentation can be used to identify areas of interest, pathology, or normal anatomy. Current methods of segmentation require either individual labor and expertise or computer program processing utilizing normal atlas templates to serve as a guide to identification of structures. Both methods are less than ideal in efficiency and accuracy. Machine learning models can be applied to normal anatomy segmentation and labeling, serving as an educational resource or reference during study interpretation. Machine learning and deep learning segmentation methods also have been applied to multiple areas in head and neck radiation treatment planning, specifically with segmentation of anatomy to assist with identifying organs at risk with treatment.[30–32] Applying intelligent segmentation of abnormal tissue in the head and neck allows for quicker quantification of lesion

characteristics, such as dimensions, volumes, texture analysis, or changes from prior examinations. Deep learning applications have shown early promise in segmentation of tumor volumes in nasopharyngeal carcinoma,[33] detecting head and neck nodal metastasis, and identifying extranodal extension of tumor.[34]

Head and neck cancer radiomics
With ever-increasing image resolution, each study of the head and neck contains a large amount of extractable information. High-level quantitative evaluation of pathologic lesions can be performed by extracting characteristics that may be invisible to the human perception, such as shape, intensity, and texture. Radiomics is the application of these imaging quantifications to biologically and clinically important characteristics of tumors, such as molecular markers and clinical behavior.[35] The amount of data and processing required for radiomic evaluation is well situated for machine learning. Du and colleagues[36] recently published work on the extraction of 525 radiomics features from MR images of nasopharyngeal carcinoma together with 5 clinical features, with the machine learning model accurately predicting 3-year disease progression. A group at MD Anderson Cancer Center evaluated radiomic features of oropharyngeal carcinoma and found the machine learning–generated radiomic signature was better at predicting recurrence after radiotherapy than clinical features, such as human papillomavirus status, smoking, and age.[37] Another recent study

applied machine learning to texture analysis of squamous cell carcinomas in the head and neck on dual-energy CT and accurately predicted the presence of nodal metastases based the primary tumor imaging characteristics.[38]

Thyroid nodule characterization

Feasibility studies on thyroid nodule detection and characterization using machine learning techniques have shown promise. Computer-aided diagnosis of benign versus malignant thyroid nodules on ultrasound images using a machine learning platform demonstrated an accuracy slightly greater than human interpretation.[39] Another recent study applied machine learning to CT images prior to thyroidectomy and trained the imaging characteristics of thyroid nodules to common immunohistochemical markers. The model demonstrated more than 80% accuracy for predicting thyroperoxidase, galectin-3, and cytokeratin-19 based on the preoperative CT.[40]

Detection of osteomeatal complex inflammation

Sinonasal inflammatory disease or rhinosinusitis frequently is imaged with CT. In chronic or recurrent rhinosinusitis, multiple repeat imaging studies often are performed throughout a patient's life. This results in a large volume of sinonasal imaging data, including longitudinal imaging data in a chronic disease state. This sinonasal imaging data repository is a prime source of information to study the correlation of imaging findings and the clinical disease. Extracting the imaging data for research purposes, however, is a time-consuming process and results in at least some interobserver disagreement. Specifically, sinonasal imaging contains complex anatomy with individual unique anatomic variations, resulting in even greater difficulty in agreement. Chowdhury and colleagues[41] applied a deep learning model to axial and coronal CT images of sinonasal inflammatory disease and trained the model to predict the osteomeatal complex as open or closed. The proof-of-concept model achieved 85% classification accuracy. With further improvement of this and similar models, a large volume of imaging studies can be processed with automated extraction of focused imaging findings and result in higher-quality statistical analysis in clinical research utilizing imaging data points.

CHALLENGES OF ARTIFICIAL INTELLIGENCE

AI in radiology is a rapidly progressing field and will become a large part of radiologists' future. Significant barriers and challenges need to be addressed, however, prior to the widespread adoption and integration of AI into clinical workflows.

Among the largest challenges to machine learning and deep learning methods are the quality, amount, and biases of the data used to train and validate the models. Ground truth labels are essential in supervised training of machine learning algorithms and absolute ground truth can be difficult to achieve. A common source of ground truth is human labeling of data. This labeling process can be subjective or susceptible to expert disagreement. For example, radiologists using the standardized American College of Radiology Thyroid Imaging, Reporting and Data System lexicon to assign features to thyroid nodules on ultrasound demonstrated only fair to moderate agreement in labeling of features.[42] This variation in labels could lead to bias with a machine learning model, and the model could be neither accurate nor generalizable for use outside its training environment. Additionally, labeling data sets requires substantial time and validation. Training systems to classify rare findings require a larger amount of data and high human time/capital cost compared with more common findings.[29] Bias also is a significant challenge to learning models. Randomized clinical trials are ideal testing environments where subjects and data are identified and collected in a prospective and controlled fashion to accurately represent the clinical scenario. Frequently, the AI models are built using retrospective and heterogenous data. This practice can lead to sampling errors and bias in the final model. In a nonradiology example, facial recognition algorithms, operating on similar machine learning programs to those discussed previously, have demonstrated elevated levels of error when assessing faces of black individuals compared with white individuals.[43] Bias in models results in poor generalizability and will be one of the largest barriers to overcome for widespread adoption.

Integration of AI into clinical operations and workflow is a significant challenge. Clinical imaging volume continues to rise year after year with high demand for radiologists to maximize productivity. Although the benefit of efficient and accurate AI would be optimal in this environment, the current state of AI applications can be disruptive to the clinical workflow. Early use and development of AI require validation because new environments can lead to unpredictable results, with supervised learning methods requiring feedback to improve. The validation of findings is an additional step in workflow and could lead to poor adoption due to the initial decrease in workflow efficiency. Large heterogeneity and widespread lack in interoperability in technical equipment, software, protocols, and picture archiving and communication systems also present significant challenges to the widespread adoption of imaging AI.

AI applications in medicine also face regulation, ethical, and legal challenges. The Food and Drug Administration provides regulation for traditional health care innovations to protect public health and safety in the United States. The traditional regulatory pathway approves devices or software prior to market introduction and can approve future modifications of previously approved products. Regulation of AI and machine learning in medicine provides unique and novel challenges as the models will continually adapt and change their operation to optimize outputs and, therefore, potentially change the results from what initially was approved. Improved transparency and real-world monitoring of software will be necessary to ensure safety. A central pillar to patient safety is protecting personal health information. Although protected health information can be scrubbed from imaging data in traditional ways prior to model training, development, or validation, powerful machine learning algorithms can extract identifiable data from images that human perception cannot. Of interest to head and neck imaging, CT and MR imaging often provide multiplanar information of individuals' faces. Facial recognition software has shown the ability to identify specific individuals based on the extraction of facial features within medical images.[44] Questions also surround liability and AI applications. In the event of an unwarranted and unjust medical outcome where AI was utilized, it currently is not clear who bears liability: the provider using the AI data, the health organization approving the use of the AI application, or the developer of the application. This question will evolve and clarify over time, but in the short term, fear of potential liability may limit adoption of new and emerging AI applications.

Lastly, AI and machine learning historically has operated as a black box. Health care decisions traditionally are well reasoned and explainable. The features extracted, weights, and decisions leading to a final output in machine learning application often are not evident and hidden. The data are provided to the model, the model undertakes processing and decision making within the black box, and the model reveals the final output only to the user. Even when the AI internal processes are understood, the technical details are complex and often cannot be explained simply to the end user, patient, or regulatory bodies. Traditional medical and scientific beliefs often require detailed understanding on how processes work, and individuals are taught to not accept information blindly if reasoning behind the information cannot be provided. Improved understanding of how machine and deep learning processes work will improve adoption into the medical arena.

SUMMARY

AI, specifically machine learning and deep learning models, are being applied rapidly to almost every aspect of imaging, including acquisition, postprocessing, worklist prioritization, interpretation, reporting, quality improvement, and research. Applications are nearly endless throughout all subfields of imaging, with head and neck imaging no different. Head and neck radiology can and should be a leader in the clinical development and application of AI, given the relative abundance of histopathologic correlation to imaging findings as well as opportunities for technologic improvement of imaging and interpretation of challenging and complex anatomy. Although AI is in its infancy for clinical integration, those who are familiar and open to the technologies while understanding the barriers and limitations will be the ones to lead the field of radiology into the future.

DISCLOSURE

The authors have nothing to disclose.

REFERENCES

1. Thrall J, Li X, Li Q, et al. Artificial intelligence and machine learning in radiology: opportunities, challenges, pitfalls, and criteria for success. J Am Coll Radiol 2016;15(26):504–8.
2. Noguerol T, Paulano-Godino F, Martín-Valdivia M, et al. Strengths, weaknesses, opportunities, and threats analysis of artificial intelligence and machine learning applications in radiology. J Am Coll Radiol 2019;16(9):1239–47.
3. Kohli M, Prevedello L, Filice R, et al. Implementing machine learning in radiology practice and research. Am J Roentgenol 2017;208(4):754–60.
4. Erickson B, Korfiatis P, Akkus Z, et al. Machine learning for medical imaging. Radiographics 2017; 37(2):505–15.
5. Chartrand G, Cheng P, Vorontsov E, et al. Deep learning: a primer for radiologists. Radiographics 2017;37(7):2113–31.
6. Obermeyer Z, Emanuel E. Predicting the future — big data, machine learning, and clinical medicine. N Engl J Med 2016;375(13):1216–9.
7. Susskind R, Susskind D. Technology will replace many doctors, lawyers, and other professionals. In: Harvard business review. 2016. Available at: https://

hbr.org/2016/10/robots-will-replace-doctors-lawyers-and-other-professionals. Accessed January 27, 2020.

8. Morgenstern M. Automation and anxiety. In: economist. 2016. Available at: https://www.economist.com/special-report/2016/06/23/automation-and-anxiety. Accessed January 27, 2020.

9. Creative Destruction Lab. Geoff Hinton: On radiology. YouTube video. 2016. Available at: https://www.youtube.com/watch?v=2HMPRXstSvQ. Accessed January 26, 2020.

10. Hinton G. Deep learning—a technology with the potential to transform health care. JAMA 2018;320(11):1101.

11. Koktzoglou I, Huang R, Ong A, et al. Feasibility of a sub-3-minute imaging strategy for ungated quiescent interval slice-selective MRA of the extracranial carotid arteries using radial k-space sampling and deep learning–based image processing. Magn Reson Med 2020;84(2):825–37.

12. Zhu G, Jiang B, Tong L, et al. Applications of deep learning to neuro-imaging techniques. Front Neurol 2019;10:869.

13. Golkov V, Dosovitskiy A, Sperl J, et al. q-Space deep learning: twelve-fold shorter and model-free diffusion MRI scans. IEEE Trans Med Imaging 2016; 35(5):1344–51.

14. Hyun C, Kim H, Lee S, et al. Deep learning for under-sampled MRI reconstruction. Phys Med Biol 2018; 63(13):135007.

15. Lee D, Yoo J, Tak S, et al. Deep residual learning for accelerated MRI using magnitude and phase networks. IEEE Trans Biomed Eng 2018;65(9):1985–95.

16. Xie S, Zheng X, Chen Y, et al. Artifact removal using improved GoogLeNet for sparse-view CT reconstruction. Sci Rep 2018;8(1):6700.

17. Chen H, Zhang Y, Kalra M, et al. Low-dose CT with a residual encoder-decoder convolutional neural network. IEEE Trans Med Imaging 2017;36(12): 2524–35.

18. Gong E, Pauly J, Wintermark M, et al. Deep learning enables reduced gadolinium dose for contrast-enhanced brain MRI. J Magn Reson Imaging 2018; 48(2):330–40.

19. Duong M, Rudie J, Wang J, et al. Convolutional neural network for automated FLAIR lesion segmentation on clinical brain MR imaging. Am J Neuroradiol 2019;40(8):1282–90.

20. Lotan E, Jain R, Razavian N, et al. State of the art: machine learning applications in glioma imaging. Am J Roentgenol 2019;212(1):26–37.

21. Fan G, Liu H, Wu Z, et al. Deep learning–based automatic segmentation of lumbosacral nerves on CT for spinal intervention: a translational study. Am J Neuroradiol 2019;40(6):1074–81.

22. Oakden-Rayner L. The rebirth of CAD: how is modern AI different from the CAD we know? Radiol Artif Intell 2019;1(3):e180089.

23. Kuo W, Häne C, Mukherjee P, et al. Expert-level detection of acute intracranial hemorrhage on head computed tomography using deep learning. Proc Natl Acad Sci U S A 2019;116(45):22737–45.

24. Sreekumari A, Shanbhag D, Yeo D, et al. A deep learning–based approach to reduce rescan and recall rates in clinical MRI examinations. Am J Neuroradiol 2019;40(2):217–23.

25. Tamada D, Kromrey M, Ichikawa S, et al. Motion artifact reduction using a convolutional neural network for dynamic contrast enhanced MR imaging of the liver. Magn Reson Med Sci 2020;19(1):64–76.

26. Haskell M, Cauley S, Bilgic B, et al. Network Accelerated Motion Estimation and Reduction (NAMER): convolutional neural network guided retrospective motion correction using a separable motion model. Magn Reson Med 2019;82(4):1452–61.

27. Cheng L, Zheng J, Savova G, et al. Discerning tumor status from unstructured MRI reports—completeness of information in existing reports and utility of automated natural language processing. J Digit Imaging 2009;23(2):119–32.

28. Lou R, Lalevic D, Chambers C, et al. Automated detection of radiology reports that require follow-up imaging using natural language processing feature engineering and machine learning classification. J Digit Imaging 2019;33(1):131–6.

29. Choy G, Khalilzadeh O, Michalski M, et al. Current applications and future impact of machine learning in radiology. Radiology 2018;288(2):318–28.

30. Zhu W, Huang Y, Zeng L, et al. AnatomyNet: deep learning for fast and fully automated whole-volume segmentation of head and neck anatomy. Med Phys 2018;46(2):579–89.

31. Kearney V, Chan J, Valdes G, et al. The application of artificial intelligence in the IMRT planning process for head and neck cancer. Oral Oncol 2018;87: 111–6.

32. Doshi T, Wilson C, Paterson C, et al. Validation of a magnetic resonance imaging-based auto-contouring software tool for gross tumour delineation in head and neck cancer radiotherapy planning. Clin Oncol 2017;29(1):60–7.

33. Lin L, Dou Q, Jin Y, et al. Deep learning for automated contouring of primary tumor volumes by MRI for nasopharyngeal carcinoma. Radiology 2019;291(3):677–86.

34. Kann B, Aneja S, Loganadane G, et al. Pretreatment identification of head and neck cancer nodal metastasis and extranodal extension using deep learning neural networks. Sci Rep 2018;8(1):14036.

35. Giraud P, Giraud P, Gasnier A, et al. Radiomics and machine learning for radiotherapy in head and neck cancers. Front Oncol 2019;9:174.

36. Du R, Lee V, Yuan H, et al. Radiomics model to predict early progression of nonmetastatic nasopharyngeal carcinoma after intensity modulation radiation

therapy: a multicenter study. Radiol Artif Intell 2019; 1(4):e180075.

37. M. D. Anderson Cancer Center Head and Neck Quantitative Imaging Working Group. Investigation of radiomic signatures for local recurrence using primary tumor texture analysis in oropharyngeal head and neck cancer patients. Sci Rep 2018; 8(1):1524.

38. Forghani R, Chatterjee A, Reinhold C, et al. Head and neck squamous cell carcinoma: prediction of cervical lymph node metastasis by dual-energy CT texture analysis with machine learning. Eur Radiol 2019;29(11):6172–81.

39. Chang Y, Paul A, Kim N, et al. Computer-aided diagnosis for classifying benign versus malignant thyroid nodules based on ultrasound images: A comparison with radiologist-based assessments. Med Phys 2019;43(1):554–67.

40. Gu J, Zhu J, Qiu Q, et al. Prediction of immunohistochemistry of suspected thyroid nodules by use of machine learning–based radiomics. Am J Roentgenol 2019;213(6):1348–57.

41. Chowdhury N, Smith T, Chandra R, et al. Automated classification of osteomeatal complex inflammation on computed tomography using convolutional neural networks. Int Forum Allergy Rhinol 2019;9(1): 46–52.

42. Hoang J, Middleton W, Farjat A, et al. Interobserver variability of sonographic features used in the american college of radiology thyroid imaging reporting and data system. Am J Roentgenol 2018;211(1): 162–7.

43. Simonite T. The best algorithms struggle to recognize black faces equally. In: Wired. Available at: https://www.wired.com/story/best-algorithms-struggle-recognize-black-faces-equally/. Accessed February 4, 2020.

44. Prior F, Brunsden B, Hildebolt C, et al. Facial recognition from volume-rendered magnetic resonance imaging data. IEEE Trans Inf Technol Biomed 2009;13(1):5–9.

Neck Imaging Reporting and Data System
Principles and Implementation

Derek Hsu, MD[a],*, Amy F. Juliano, MD[b]

KEYWORDS

- Neck imaging reporting and data system • NI-RADS • Standardized reporting • Reporting template
- Cancer surveillance • Head and neck cancer

KEY POINTS

- The Neck Imaging Reporting and Data System (NI-RADS) is a standardized reporting template for posttreatment surveillance in head and neck cancer.
- NI-RADS assigns a numerical category, ranging from 0 to 4, one to the primary tumor site and one to the neck, each conveying the level of suspicion for tumor and linked recommended management.
- This article reviews the goals of NI-RADS, NI-RADS categories and lexicon, current research, and the future direction of NI-RADS in posttreatment head and neck cancer surveillance.

INTRODUCTION

Head and neck squamous cell carcinoma (HNSCC) represents approximately 3.7% of new cancer cases in 2019 in the United States.[1] Clinical management of these patients is complex and often includes multiple surgeries, radiation therapy, and chemotherapy. Even after completing initial treatment, HNSCC patients face considerable morbidity. Otolaryngologists can visualize superficial mucosal disease on physical examination and endoscopy. Radiologists play an integral role in cancer surveillance because they are able to identify deep abnormalities.

Currently there is no standardized HNSCC posttreatment surveillance imaging algorithm, leading to variability between institutions and clinicians. The 2019 National Comprehensive Cancer Network guidelines are not specific.[2] For surveillance, it recommends consideration of imaging within 6 months of treatment completion. Any imaging beyond 6 months is completely reliant on the discretion of the physician and the clinical suspicion. Annual imaging surveillance may only be indicated if an area is "difficult to visualize on physical exam."[2] In addition, concrete, longer-term posttreatment imaging recommendations and guidelines, such as choice of imaging modality and time intervals, remain absent.

In recent years, standardized reporting with reporting templates and linked management guidelines, or Reporting and Data System (RADS), has gained traction in radiology. The development of RADS began as an initiative by the American College of Radiology (ACR) to decrease interobserver report variability among radiologists and to deliver care that is "patient-centric, data-driven, and outcomes-based."[3] Each RADS is modality specific, pertains to a specific disease process, and contains several components: standardized terminology, or "lexicon" as descriptors of imaging findings, a

[a] Department of Radiology and Imaging Sciences, Emory University School of Medicine, 1364 Clifton Road Northeast, Suite BG03, Atlanta, GA 30322, USA; [b] Department of Radiology, Massachusetts Eye and Ear, Harvard Medical School, 243 Charles Street, Boston, MA 02114, USA
* Corresponding author.
E-mail address: derek.evan.hsu@emory.edu
Twitter: @amyfjuliano (A.F.J.)

Neuroimag Clin N Am 30 (2020) 369–377
https://doi.org/10.1016/j.nic.2020.05.001
1052-5149/20/© 2020 Elsevier Inc. All rights reserved.

neuroimaging.theclinics.com

recommended reporting template, and numerical categories that denote the probability of disease occurrence. The first RADS that came into being was the Breast Imaging Reporting and Data System or BI-RADS, developed for mammography for detection of breast cancer. Subsequently, other systems followed, including TI-RADS for thyroid nodule imaging, LI-RADS for hepatocellular carcinoma imaging, Lung-RADS for lung cancer screening, and PI-RADS for prostate cancer imaging.

The purpose of this article is to review the goals, classification and lexicon, current research, and future direction of Neck Imaging Reporting and Data System (NI-RADS) for posttreatment head and neck cancer surveillance.

AMERICAN COLLEGE OF RADIOLOGY NECK IMAGING REPORTING AND DATA SYSTEM OVERVIEW

Interpretation of posttreatment HNSCC surveillance imaging poses a challenge to many radiologists because of anatomic complexity and its often distorted posttreatment appearance. The neck is a relatively compact area of the body with intricate anatomy, containing many critical neurovascular structures and almost half of the body's lymph nodes. Patients may undergo extensive surgical resections with various composite free-flap reconstructions, altering anatomic architecture and rendering radiologic interpretation challenging to those radiologists who are not accustomed to these cases. In the setting of chemoradiation therapy (CRT), treatment-related soft tissue swelling and contrast enhancement from edema, inflammation, or granulation tissue may be mistaken for recurrent tumor.[4]

In response to these challenges, a committee comprising head and neck radiologists from multiple academic centers across the country developed the ACR NI-RADS. NI-RADS was originally designed for use in the setting of surveillance imaging after treated HNSCC for contrast-enhanced computed tomography (CECT), with or without fluorodeoxyglucose (FDG) PET. At its inception, the NI-RADS committee had the following goals:

1. Create standardized imaging terminology or lexicon for head and neck masses in order to differentiate benign from malignant.
2. By using the lexicon, develop a risk-stratified classification system to clearly communicate to referring clinicians which head and neck masses require short-term follow-up or immediate biopsy.

3. Generate data-mineable reports to help assess and refine surveillance algorithms, improve accuracy, and decrease interobserver variability.

Historically, posttreatment HNSCC surveillance radiology reports were free-form without specific organization or structure. If the radiologist's report is not explicit in committing to a disease status, it places the onus on the referring clinician to interpret the radiologist's suspicion for the presence of disease. By adopting a standardized lexicon and structured report, radiologists are encouraged to communicate their imaging assessment using uniform, unambiguous language and assign a risk-stratified numerical category. With this numerical category, referring clinicians can easily and unambiguously determine the next recommended step in management.

The adoption of NI-RADS provides an avenue to retrospectively evaluate interobserver variability and reveal potential common pitfalls among radiologists. In turn, this allows for the creation of educational material and improvement of radiologist accuracy. In addition, by examining patient outcomes, NI-RADS provides a foundation to help guide the ongoing improvement and evolution of an optimal standardized surveillance algorithm. The ultimate goal in instituting NI-RADS is to improve patient care and optimize quality of life for patients with head and neck cancer.

NECK IMAGING REPORTING AND DATA SYSTEM CATEGORIES AND LEXICON

Use of a standardized classification system and lexicon is integral to NI-RADS. In posttreatment surveillance of HNSCC, the primary tumor site and lymph node or neck site are evaluated for locally residual or recurrent disease and for metastatic adenopathy. Each site is assigned a NI-RADS numerical category independently, which conveys a specific level of suspicion for the presence of disease. This numerical category ranges from 0 through 4: (0) incomplete, (1) no evidence of local recurrence (primary site) or adenopathy (neck), (2) low suspicion, (3) high suspicion, and (4) definite recurrence. Each NI-RADS category has its own specific lexicon and linked management, as shown in **Table 1**.

Neck Imaging Reporting and Data System 0: Incomplete

A NI-RADS category 0 is assigned to a new baseline study with prior imaging that is not yet available to the radiologist but will be made available in the future. When the comparison study becomes available, a NI-RADS category may be

Table 1
Neck Imaging Reporting and Data System categories and descriptors

Category	Primary Site	Primary Imaging Findings	Neck Site	Neck Imaging Findings	Management
Incomplete	0	• New baseline study with prior imaging that is not available, but will become available as comparison in the future	0	• New baseline study with prior imaging that is not available, but will become available as comparison in the future	Assign category in an addendum after prior imaging examinations become available
No evidence of recurrence	1	• Expected posttreatment appearance • Non-masslike distortion of soft tissues • Low-density posttreatment mucosal edema • Diffuse, curvilinear mucosal enhancement or FDG uptake • No abnormal FDG uptake	1	• Expected posttreatment appearance • No FDG uptake in residual nodal tissue	Routine surveillance
Low suspicion	2a	Mucosal: • Focal mucosal enhancement or FDG uptake on initial posttreatment scan	2	• Mild/moderate FDG uptake in residual nodal tissue • Enlarging or new lymph node without definitive abnormal morphologic features [b] • Discrepancy between PET and CECT: 1. Enlarging lymph node or discrete neck mass with little to no FDG uptake 2. Focal FDG uptake without CECT correlate	2a: Direct visual inspection
Low suspicion	2b	Deep: • Ill-defined soft tissue with only mild/moderate FDG uptake if PET available • Discrepancy between PET and CECT: 1. Discrete CECT abnormality with little to no FDG uptake [a] 2. Focal FDG uptake without CECT correlate			2b or neck 2: short-interval follow-up

(continued on next page)

Table 1
(continued)

Category	Primary Site	Primary Imaging Findings	Neck Site	Neck Imaging Findings	Management

High suspicion	3	• Discrete nodule or mass at the primary tumor site with intense focal FDG uptake	3	• Residual nodal tissue with intense FDG uptake
				• New enlarged or enlarging lymph node with:
				  1. Abnormal morphologic features
				  2. Focal intense FDG uptake
					Biopsy if clinically indicated

Definitive recurrence	4	• Pathologically proven tumor or definite radiologic or clinical progression of disease	4	• Pathologically proven tumor or definite radiologic or clinical progression of disease	Clinical management

[a] Only if the original tumor was FDG-avid.

[b] New necrosis or gross extranodal extension as evidenced by invasion of adjacent structures.

Adapted from American College of Radiology. NI-RADS Category Descriptors, Imaging Findings, and Management. Published 2019. Accessed January 4, 2019. https://www.acr.org/-/media/ACR/Files/RADS/NI-RADS/NIRADS-Category-Descriptors.pdf.

assigned in an addendum at that time. If prior imaging exists but to the knowledge of the radiologist will not be made available, then a NI-RADS 0 cannot be assigned. Instead, an appropriate category must be determined by the radiologist with the available data.

Neck Imaging Reporting and Data System 1: No Evidence of Recurrence

A NI-RADS category 1 represents an imaging study with benign findings and expected post-treatment changes. Lexicon and imaging appearance of this category are as follows:

- Expected posttreatment changes
- No abnormal FDG uptake
- Non-masslike soft tissue distortion without a discrete mass
- Mucosal findings:
  - Low-density submucosal edema (most likely postradiation)
  - Diffuse curvilinear enhancement or FDG uptake (most likely radiation-induced mucositis)
- Residual lymph node tissue without FDG avidity

The recommended management is routine surveillance imaging. A common time interval until the next scan is 6 months, but may be tailored as specific to the individual practice's surveillance algorithm.

Neck Imaging Reporting and Data System 2: Low Suspicion

A NI-RADS category 2 represents an imaging study that is indeterminate for disease, with an imaging finding that most likely represents posttreatment change, although tumor recurrence remains a consideration. Lexicon and imaging appearance of a NI-RADS 2 are as follows:

- Focal mucosal enhancement or FDG uptake on initial posttreatment scan
- Deep, ill-defined soft tissue, and with only mild to moderate FDG uptake if a PET is available
- Any discordance between PET and CECT:
  - A discrete CECT abnormality with little to no FDG uptake (this applies only if the original tumor was FDG-avid before treatment)
  - Focal FDG uptake without CECT correlate
- Mild to moderate FDG uptake in residual lymph node tissue
- Enlarging or new lymph node without definitive abnormal morphologic features, such as new necrosis or extranodal extension

In the case of an indeterminate lesion, short-term radiologic or clinical evaluation is needed. If it is a superficial abnormality (NI-RADS 2a), direct visual inspection is recommended. If instead a deep abnormality is present (NI-RADS 2b), short-interval follow-up imaging with CECT or PET in 3 months is recommended.

Neck Imaging Reporting and Data System 3: High Suspicion

A NI-RADS category 3 represents a study that contains imaging findings that are highly suspicious for residual or recurrent tumor (**Figs. 1** and **2**). Lexicon and imaging appearance of NI-RADS 3 are as follows:

- A discrete nodule or mass at the primary site with intense contrast enhancement, or focal FDG uptake if a PET is available
- Residual lymph node tissue with intense FDG uptake
- A new enlarged lymph node or progressively enlarging lymph node with abnormal morphologic features on CECT, such as new necrosis or extranodal extension, or focal intense FDG uptake if a PET is available

In order to confirm or exclude the presence of residual or recurrent tumor, the recommended next management step is immediate biopsy of the imaging abnormality.

Neck Imaging Reporting and Data System 4: Definite Recurrence

A NI-RADS category 4 is assigned to patients with either pathology-proven recurrence or definite radiologic or clinical progression of disease (**Fig. 3**). Radiologically, the Response Evaluation Criteria in Solid Tumors (RECIST) criteria[5] help guide radiologists when tumor is worsening. The recommended management is clinical management with or without a biopsy.

IMPLEMENTATION OF NECK IMAGING REPORTING AND DATA SYSTEM AND RESULTS

Adoption of NI-RADS is relatively easy because all NI-RADS information can be easily accessed online through the ACR Web site (https://www.acr.org/Clinical-Resources/Reporting-and-Data-Systems/NI-RADs). The Web site provides training and education resources to help launch NI-RADS utilization in daily clinical reporting, including a NI-RADS atlas, which provides a brief background, and most importantly, sample clinical cases for review. Also available is a suggested

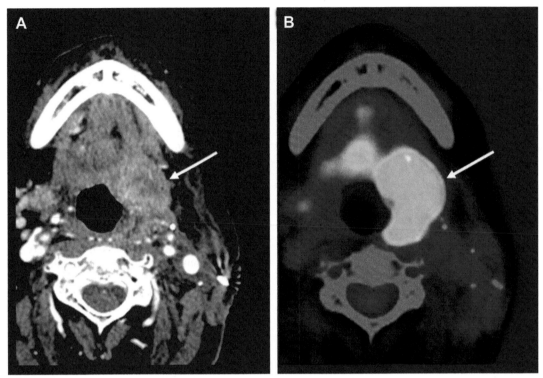

Fig. 1. Primary site NI-RADS 3 on PET/CECT: a patient with a history of left oral tongue squamous cell carcinoma treated with left hemiglossectomy, selective neck dissection, radial forearm free-flap reconstruction, and CRT. Posttreatment surveillance PET/CECT demonstrates a new, heterogeneously enhancing, bulky soft tissue lesion (*arrow* in A) with intense FDG uptake (*arrow* in B) along the left base of tongue extending toward the floor of mouth and parapharyngeal space deep to the flap. As a result of this highly suspicious finding, a biopsy of the lesion was performed, confirming recurrent squamous cell carcinoma.

reporting template and surveillance legend. The legend provides a short description of each numerical category and the associated recommended management.

Performance of NI-RADS has been examined in several published retrospective studies. In the initial Krieger and colleagues[6] NI-RADS study, 500 consecutive neck CECTs from 2014 to 2015 were reported using the NI-RADS template; of those, 318 studies and 618 targets (314 primary tumor site targets and 304 neck site targets) met inclusion and exclusion criteria. Residual and recurrent disease was confirmed by a positive biopsy of a suspicious imaging finding; definite radiologic progression was determined per RECIST criteria or clear clinical progression on physical examination. Most surveillance studies were categorized as NI-RADS 1: 85.4% (528 targets of 618 targets), among which the recurrence rate was 3.8% (20/528). Fewer were categorized as NI-RADS 2, 19.4% (58 targets of 618 targets), among which the recurrence rate was 17.2% (10/58). The fewest number of studies were categorized as NI-RADS 3, 5.2% (32 targets of the 618

targets), among which the recurrence rate was 59.4% (19/32). NI-RADS 4 was not included in the analysis, because they represent 100% disease recurrence by definition. The investigators demonstrated a statistically significant association between NI-RADS score and disease recurrence at the primary, neck, and combined primary and neck sites.[6]

Although the initial study examined all surveillance time points with NI-RADS reporting, subsequent studies focused on only the first posttreatment time point, typically 2 to 3 months after treatment completion. In Hsu and colleagues,[7] all first posttreatment PET/CECTs scans between 2014 and 2016 were collected, excluding all other time points. There was a similar distribution of NI-RADS categories and recurrence rates in the included 199 scans or 397 targets (108 primary targets and 109 nodal targets). NI-RADS 1 again represented most of the cohort, 75.8% (301 targets of 397 targets), and had a recurrence rate of 4.3% (13/301). NI-RADS 2 represented 19.4% of the cohort (77 targets of 397 targets) and had a recurrence rate of

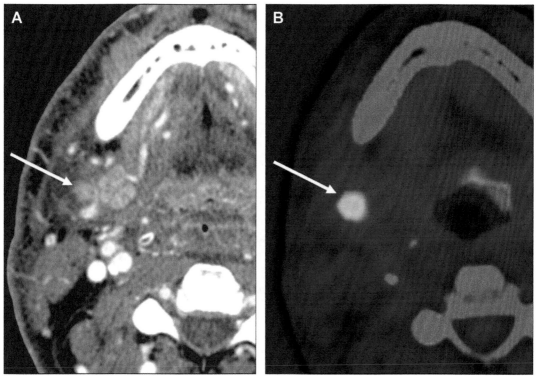

Fig. 2. Neck/node NI-RADS 3 on PET/CECT: a patient with a history of right tonsillar squamous cell carcinoma treated with CRT. Posttreatment baseline surveillance PET/CECT demonstrates a 7-mm nodule in the right submandibular region (*arrow* in *A*) with intense FDG uptake (*arrow* in *B*). The patient elected for a repeat PET/CECT in 3 months, which demonstrated resolution of this finding.

9.1% (7/77). Again, NI-RADS 3 represented the smallest percentage of the cohort, 4.8% (19 targets of 397 targets), and had a recurrence rate of 42.1% (8/19). The investigators demonstrated that a higher NI-RADS score is significantly associated with increasing risk for treatment failure at both the primary and neck sites (hazards ratio: 2.6 and 5.2, respectively).

Interestingly, in a small subgroup analysis of the Hsu and colleagues[7] study, a higher NI-RADS score did not demonstrate a statistically significant association with treatment failure at the primary site in patients who were surgically treated with or without CRT. These data should be interpreted with caution, however, because this was an extremely small cohort (90 patients). Further studies are needed to examine how different treatment modalities may influence NI-RADS score in the posttreatment setting.

Previous data reported a negative predictive value (NPV) of 91% for negative PET/CECT or NI-RADS 1.[8] Wangaryattawanich and colleagues[9] examined the NI-RADS 2 category, specifically those patients with incomplete/partial treatment response. A total of 2077 patients

had a first posttreatment PET/CECT between 2008 and 2016. Each patient's study was reviewed to determine whether it met criteria for NI-RADS 2: a decrease in tumor size or FDG avidity but persistent mild FDG uptake or residual soft tissue at the primary or neck site. Twenty-two percent (464/2077) of patients met criteria for NI-RADS 2. Of these 464 patients, 110 patients met inclusion and exclusion criteria. A total of 17 patients were determined to have locoregional treatment failure within 2 years, or a recurrence rate of 15% (17/110), yielding an NPV of 85% at the first posttreatment scan. The investigators concluded that patients with an initial incomplete response (NI-RADS 2) require more frequent and shorter-term follow-up than for patients with an initial complete response (NI-RADS 1).

These retrospective studies using the NI-RADS template demonstrate its utility and value in posttreatment surveillance PET/CECT in HNSCC patients. NI-RADS 1 represented the most population with the lowest recurrence rate. With each subsequent stepwise increase in NI-RADS category, there was an increasingly higher rate

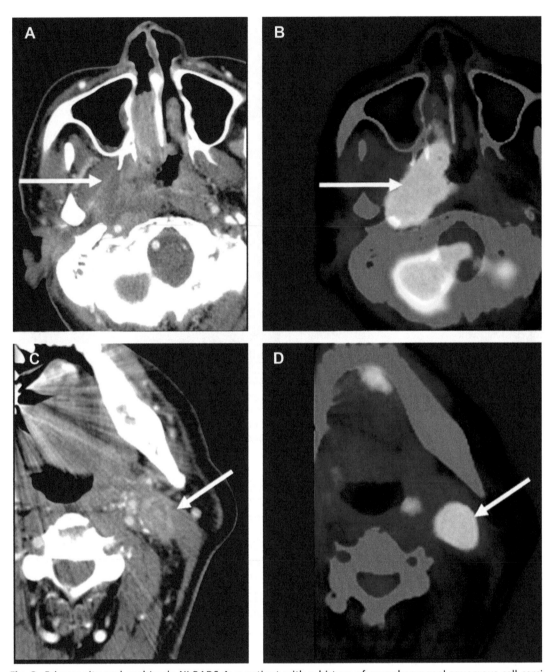

Fig. 3. Primary site and neck/node NI-RADS 4: a patient with a history of nasopharyngeal squamous cell carcinoma treated with CRT. Posttreatment baseline surveillance PET/CECT demonstrates the presence of tumor at the primary site and the neck site. (*A, B*) Residual mass is seen extensively involving the right nasopharyngeal region and masticator space (*arrow* in *A*) with associated intense FDG avidity (*arrow* in *B*). There is also extensive bone erosion (not shown). (*C, D*) A left level II node is abnormally large and heterogeneously enhancing (*arrow* in *C*), with intense FDG avidity (*arrow* in *D*).

of recurrence while representing a smaller percentage of the population (Table 2). By adopting NI-RADS, clinicians may provide concrete data on the probability of tumor to patients when reviewing radiology findings and reports.

FUTURE DIRECTION OF NECK IMAGING REPORTING AND DATA SYSTEM

Posttreatment evaluation of HNSCC is most often accomplished with CECT with or without

Table 2
Reported prevalence and recurrence rate of Neck Imaging Reporting and Data System

NI-RADS Category	Prevalence			Recurrence Rate		
	Krieger et al,[6] 2017, %	Wangaryattawanich et al,[9] 2018, %	Hsu et al,[7] 2019, %	Krieger et al,[6] 2017, %	Wangaryattawanich et al,[9] 2018, %	Hsu et al,[7] 2019, %
NI-RADS 1	85.4	—	75.8	3.8	—	4.3
NI-RADS 2	9.4	22	19.4	17.2	15	9.1
NI-RADS 3	5.2	—	4.8	59.4	—	42.1

PET. However, there is an important role for MR imaging in surveillance as well, either complementary to CT or as the primary modality for locations not as amenable to CT assessment. For instance, MR imaging is particularly good at detecting laryngeal cartilage invasion and is the preferred modality for assessment of the sinonasal cavities and skull base, and for assessment of perineural spread of tumor.[10] As such, an MR image–specific NI-RADS reporting template with associated lexicon is currently under development.

One of the major goals of NI-RADS was to reduce the interobserver variability among radiologists when evaluating these complex posttreatment surveillance studies. In the initial NI-RADS study, interobserver agreement was examined through the kappa statistic between 2 neuroradiologists from the same institution after reviewing 40 imaging studies. The results showed very good agreement, with a kappa statistic of 0.82.[6] Although the results were encouraging, additional studies are needed for comparison between radiologists with varying degrees of experience as well as exposure to different practice patterns. It is important to evaluate the degree of agreement among radiologists using NI-RADS from different parts of the country as well, as the report template becomes more widely used.

SUMMARY

Reporting templates have become an integral aspect of radiology. Complex postsurgical and post-CRT anatomic distortion of the head and neck can lead to long and ambiguous reports without any next clinical management step. By adopting NI-RADS, radiologists must commit to a category and thus convey a specific level of suspicion for residual or recurrent tumor. It is the hope that, by decreasing variability in radiology reports and clinical management, outcomes for patients with head and neck cancer ultimately improve.

DISCLOSURE

The authors have nothing to disclose.

REFERENCES

1. Siegel RL, Miller KD, Jemal A. Cancer statistics, 2019. CA Cancer J Clin 2019;69(1):7–34.
2. Network NCC. Head and neck cancer (version 3.2019). 2019. Available at: https://www.nccn.org/professionals/physician_gls/pdf/head-and-neck.pdf. Accessed January 4, 2020.
3. Aiken AH, Farley A, Baugnon KL, et al. Implementation of a novel surveillance template for head and neck cancer: neck imaging reporting and data system (NI-RADS). J Am Coll Radiol 2016;13(6):743–6.e1.
4. Taghipour M, Sheikhbahaei S, Wray R, et al. FDG PET/CT in patients with head and neck squamous cell carcinoma after primary surgical resection with or without chemoradiation therapy. AJR Am J Roentgenol 2016;206(5):1093–100.
5. Eisenhauer EA, Therasse P, Bogaerts J, et al. New response evaluation criteria in solid tumours: revised RECIST guideline (version 1.1). Eur J Cancer 2009; 45(2):228–47.
6. Krieger DA, Hudgins PA, Nayak GK, et al. Initial performance of NI-RADS to predict residual or recurrent head and neck squamous cell carcinoma. AJNR Am J Neuroradiol 2017;38(6):1193–9.
7. Hsu D, Chokshi FH, Hudgins PA, et al. Predictive value of first posttreatment imaging using standardized reporting in head and neck cancer. Otolaryngol Head Neck Surg 2019;161(6):978–85.
8. McDermott M, Hughes M, Rath T, et al. Negative predictive value of surveillance PET/CT in head and neck squamous cell cancer. AJNR Am J Neuroradiol 2013;34(8):1632–6.
9. Wangaryattawanich P, Branstetter BFT, Hughes M, et al. Negative predictive value of NI-RADS category 2 in the first posttreatment FDG-PET/CT in head and neck squamous cell carcinoma. AJNR Am J Neuroradiol 2018;39(10):1884–8.
10. Becker M, Zaidi H. Imaging in head and neck squamous cell carcinoma: the potential role of PET/MRI. Br J Radiol 2014;87(1036):20130677.

Common Data Elements in Head and Neck Radiology Reporting

Anandh G. Rajamohan, MD[a,*], Vishal Patel, MD, PhD[a,b],
Nasim Sheikh-Bahaei, MD, PhD[a], Chia-Shang J. Liu, MD, PhD[a],
John L. Go, MD[a], Paul E. Kim, MD[a], Wende Gibbs, MD[c], Jay Acharya, MD[a]

KEYWORDS

- Common data elements (CDEs) • Artificial intelligence • Informatics • Structured reporting
- Standardization • Quality improvement • Value in radiology

KEY POINTS

- Common data elements with respect to radiology reporting are standardized embeddable content that addresses specific best-practice concepts with discrete responses that can be used regardless of reporting style and with potential to be consumed by humans and machines alike.
- Although common data elements and structured reports share some similarities and benefits with traditional narrative reporting, contextual reporting and common data elements are more closely linked, offering more opportunity in the future, with common data elements having more flexibility.
- Common data elements will be a key method to train machine learning systems and incorporate clinical decision support and other patient safety and quality improvement processes.

INTRODUCTION

Head and neck imaging is a crossroad for many medical specialties, ranging from otolaryngology, radiology, pathology, oncology, radiation oncology, to primary care. The anatomy and potential pathologies are often considered to be complex, making the radiology report crucial for communicating and cataloging key information.[1] The lack of consensus on how radiologists should report these cases is one of the current obstacles to advancing clinical care, research, and quality assurance on a large scale.[2] Common data elements (CDEs) stand to be a potential bridge between differences in reporting style and provide a degree of standardization across all radiologists for any given type of imaging examination. CDEs also may ease and accelerate the transition to the use of artificial intelligence and machine learning systems to further advance radiology and the practice of head and neck imaging.

COMMON DATA ELEMENTS: DEFINITION AND EXAMPLES

A CDE is a granular concept or question with a discrete set of constrained answers for a given situation or setting. It can also be thought of as a

[a] Department of Radiology, Division of Neuroradiology, University of Southern California, Keck School of Medicine, 1500 San Pablo Street, Second Floor, Los Angeles, CA 90033, USA; [b] USC Mark and Mary Stevens Neuroimaging and Informatics Institute, University of Southern California, Keck School of Medicine, 2025 Zonal Avenue, Los Angeles, CA 90033, USA; [c] Department of Radiology, Mayo Clinic School of Medicine, 18522 North 96th Way, Scottsdale, AZ 85255, USA
* Corresponding author. Department of Radiology, 1500 San Pablo Street, Second Floor, Los Angeles, CA 90033.
E-mail address: anandh.rajamohan@med.usc.edu
Twitter: @ARajamohan (A.G.R.)

Neuroimag Clin N Am 30 (2020) 379–391
https://doi.org/10.1016/j.nic.2020.05.002
1052-5149/20/© 2020 Elsevier Inc. All rights reserved.

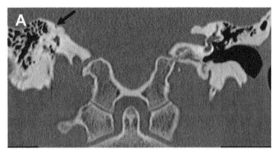
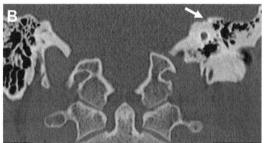

C

FINDINGS:
Left
There is absence of the bony covering of the left superior semicircular canal, best appreciated on coronal images (8:90).

The external auditory canal is patent without evidence of soft tissue mass or bony erosion. The middle ear cavity is well pneumatized without evidence of fluid or debris. All ossicles are demonstrated and unremarkable in their appearance.

The oval and round windows are identified. The cochlea demonstrates proper partitioning and the cochlear aperture is of normal width. The vestibular and cochlear aqueducts are normal in caliber. The internal auditory canal demonstrates normal morphology. The facial canal demonstrates normal course and caliber without evidence of bony dehiscence. There are a few opacified left mastoid air cells.

Right
There is marked thinning of the bone overlying the right superior semicircular canal (8:86).

The external auditory canal is patent without evidence of soft tissue mass or bony erosion. The middle ear cavity is well pneumatized without evidence of fluid or debris. All ossicles are demonstrated and unremarkable in their appearance.

The oval and round windows are identified. The cochlea demonstrates proper partitioning and the cochlear aperture is of normal width. The vestibular and cochlear aqueducts are normal in caliber. The internal auditory canal demonstrates normal morphology. The facial canal demonstrates normal course and caliber without evidence of bony dehiscence. The mastoid air cells are well pneumatized without evidence of fluid or debris.

IMPRESSION:
1. Left superior semicircular canal dehiscence.

2. Marked thinning of the right superior semicircular canal bony covering.

Fig. 1. A 35-year-old man presents with vertigo exacerbated by loud noise. (*A, B*) Coronal reformatted computed tomography (CT) images of the temporal bones without contrast show thinning of the bone covering the right superior semicircular canal (*black arrow*) and dehiscence of the left semicircular canal (*white arrow*) respectively. (*C*) These findings are conveyed in a narrative reporting style using full sentences organized into paragraphs.

"question, concept, measurement, or feature with a set of controlled responses."[3] For example, the defined responses could be quantitative (numerical value), Boolean (yes/no), defined text, or ordinal (I, II, III, IV). In the strict informatics context, a CDE is an individual piece of data.

Most radiologists encounter and use basic CDEs every day. For example, the name of a patient is an example of an identifier CDE that appears on radiology reports with the input option being text. The age of the patient is another CDE with an expected integer value. However, for the purposes of this article and use of the term CDE with respect to radiology reporting, they can be thought of as a set of related CDEs grouped together to comprise an insertable report macro or template encapsulating best-practice or essential concepts to be included in the findings or impression portion of the report.[3] These critical elements should be included for a specific examination type or context, regardless of who the interpreting radiologist is and the radiologist's preferred style of reporting.[3] CDEs should be structured information capable of being "collected and stored uniformly across institutions and studies."[4] For example, a radiologist consistently reporting details of a head and neck cancer examination in terms of the primary lesion (size, location, regional involvement), nodal disease (location, size), and presence of metastases with standardized terminology to facilitate American Joint Committee on Cancer (AJCC) tumor, node, metastasis (TNM) staging would constitute practical CDE implementation.[5,6] The emphasis on a CDE is to provide critical information in a consistent fashion to drive clinical decision making and thereby maximize the value of the radiologist, which ultimately serves to optimize patient care.

ADVANTAGES OF COMMON DATA ELEMENTS

CDEs maximize the value of the radiology report and the radiologist in the clinical care of patients by highlighting key concepts or findings in a consistent fashion. In addition, CDEs can serve as a framework that may readily facilitate future benefits through research and quality initiatives.[2] In radiology reporting, the emphasis should be on standardized reporting that will help the medical team establish diagnosis, guide therapy, and gauge treatment response. CDE information may allow for mass customization or allow researchers to integrate imaging phenotypes to support initiatives in precision medicine, allowing more patient-specific treatments.[2,7,8]

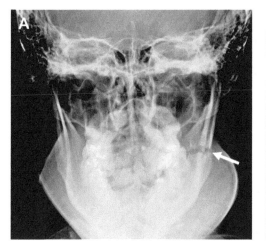
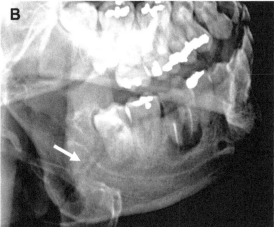
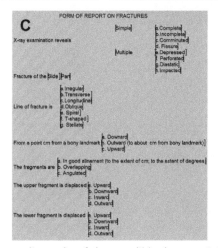

Fig. 2. (*A, B*) Frontal and oblique radiographs of the mandible show a minimally displaced fracture of the left mandibular ramus along the angle of the mandible (*white arrows*). (*C*) A literal modern translation of Preston Hickey's[24] proposed Form of Report on Fractures from his 1922 article in *American Journal of Roentgenology* follows a structured reporting format and incorporates CDEs as shown by the defined answer choices to properly describe the fracture.

By the nature of standardized discrete concepts generated from best practices and literature, CDEs should foster better patient outcomes and reduce errors from radiologists in terms of failing to communicate the most clinically relevant information by providing small internal checklists. Residents and fellows who train in practices or institutions using CDEs also stand to gain from learning about the content and purpose of CDEs.

CDEs could be used to help recruitment and capture patients for enrollment in ongoing and future clinical trials.[2,9] Because the data from CDEs are specific and shareable, this also opens the door for multicenter collaboration in research, as well through improved data registries.[10,11] Along these lines, the data are also ideal for quality improvement purposes at the individual, departmental, institutional, or national level. CDEs may also help radiology departments transition to quality-based and value-based reimbursement models, as outlined by the Merit-based Incentive Payment System and the Medicare Access and Children's Health Insurance Program Reauthorization Act.[12] In addition, one of the greatest upsides to CDEs comes from their inherent ability to be consumed and used by machine learning algorithms.[13] This ability provides annotated data for training and feedback for diagnostic systems and integration into clinical decision support software to give standard recommendations and trigger critical result reporting for better patient care.[14,15]

There are few downsides to implementing CDEs into head and neck imaging or any other radiology

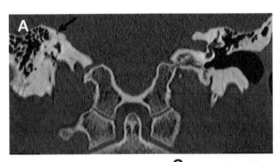
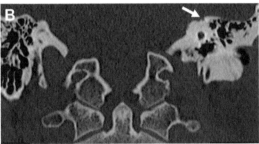
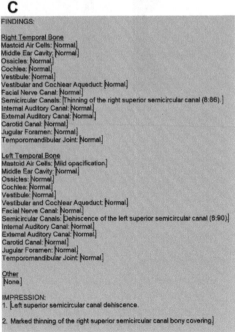

Fig. 3. A 35-year-old man presents with vertigo exacerbated by loud noise. (*A, B*) Coronal reformatted images from CT of the temporal bones without contrast show thinning of the bone covering the right superior semicircular canal (*black arrow*) and dehiscence of the left semicircular canal (*white arrow*) respectively. (*C*) A structured report is now used to depict these findings with consistently ordered and organized headings in a concise fashion.

subspecialty reporting. The time and effort required to add a CDE might be thought of as a minor negative, but an equal argument could be made that it may be saving time and is more efficient compared with a narrative dictation encompassing the same information. At present, radiologists have to be aware of and recognize the appropriate times to use CDEs and decide which CDEs are correct. Nonetheless, the authors surmise that artificial intelligence systems assisting radiologists may help automate this process in the future.

NARRATIVE REPORTING

At present, head and neck radiology reporting remains a heterogeneous landscape with each individual radiologist choosing how to describe or translate the imaging findings into a text format.[16] Typically, the terminology is chosen by the radiologist, who constructs a narrative text description of the interpretation, which is variable in length, lexicon, and style (Fig. 1).[17] The lack of standardization makes sharing, comparing, and compiling the data in these reports difficult.

In this narrative framework, the content of the report is intended to be reviewed by an ordering physician. In some situations, a portion of the language and content within the report may be generated in an attempt to limit medical liability as well.[18,19] Furthermore, radiology reports are also becoming increasingly available to be viewed by the patients.[20,21] The commonality of these 3 forces is that each is intended for human consumption.

With significant effort, the data in radiology reports can be converted into standardized information that can be used for larger-scale clinical care, research, and quality assessment. Often this requires manual review of the report by a human or discussion of the case and relevant imaging in a multidisciplinary meeting or tumor board. Effort has also been made to have computers help extract these data through natural language processing, but much of this currently has been limited to finding key words in reports or looking for pertinent negatives.[22]

STRUCTURED REPORTING

The notion of a standardized reporting format in radiology is not new and can be traced back as early as 1899 to Preston M. Hickey MD, former chairman of radiology at the University of Michigan and one of the founders of the *American Journal of Roentgenology*.[23] In his 1922 article, Hickey[24] stated that "reports submitted by a roentgenologist were inferior to those of a pathologist and were haphazard and without respect for scientific accuracy." He advocated for reports using standard nomenclature and format (Fig. 2).

The modern structured report tries to address the concerns raised by Dr Hickey[24] nearly 100 years earlier, which still plague contemporary radiology reporting: verbose reports inconsistent in organization, terminology, and content. A typical structured report includes defined headings for each core component of the report, including the clinical history/indication, comparison studies, procedure/technique, findings, and impression (Fig. 3).[25] Within the findings, there are standard subheadings for different anatomic components or disorders that might be encountered when reviewing the specific examination type at hand, or what is known as a list-style report.[25] These headings and subheadings are consistently organized and formatted. The Radiological Society of North America (RSNA) has made available more than 200 structured report templates to the public through an open library (www.radreport.org).[26] For

Table 1 Common data elements and structured reporting	
Similarities	**Differences**
Consistency in content and organization	CDE is not a complete comprehensive examination report
Concise communication of clinical information	SR does not address a specific clinical question
Facilitate trainee education	SR may provide superfluous information in the report
Billing error reduction	SR does not have a restrictive answer for each heading
Data mining and AI potential	—
Critical result reporting	—
Integration into clinical decision support systems	—
Provide systematic follow-up and recommendation	—

Abbreviations: AI, artificial intelligence; SR, structured reporting.

the head and neck, examples of headings for a computed tomography (CT) of the neck report include the suprahyoid neck, infrahyoid neck, and lymph nodes with a magnetic resonance (MR) imaging of the orbit report including headings for the globes, lacrimal glands, and extraocular muscles.[27]

The structured report requires the radiologist to address each of the heading categories, typically with a short, concise description with an emphasis on standard terminology or an accepted lexicon.[28–30] In doing so, all radiologists using the same structured report template should comment on the same anatomic areas or disorders denoted by the headings. The overall effect is a more consistent report regardless of the radiologist. The structured report also serves as a checklist and enforces consistent search patterns promoting error reduction.[31] Many clinicians find these reports easier to read and interpret.[32] Others have also shown use of structured reporting to improve with billing and efficiency in reporting.[33]

Despite concerted efforts by many radiology societies, health systems, and radiology departments to push for structured reporting, acceptance remains mixed.[34,35] Many radiologists think that structured reports are too impersonal or find them to be generic.[17,36,37] Others find that the compartmentalized format with discrete headings is difficult or restrictive to use, such as when findings cross multiple report headings.[38,39] A phenomenon known as eye dwell has also been described with structured reporting, in which the radiologist spends more time looking at the report template relative to time spent viewing the images, which can lead to errors.[18] Several studies have shown the reported benefits of structured reporting compared with prose reporting to be overstated or not necessarily present.[36]

COMMON DATA ELEMENTS VERSUS STRUCTURED REPORTING: SIMILARITIES

Both CDEs and structured reports emphasize consistency and organization in content and terminology. Both of these reporting paradigms lend themselves to concise and direct communication of clinical information. Many of the error reduction, billing, and trainee educational advantages are also shared along with data mining potential and potential for artificial intelligence consumption.

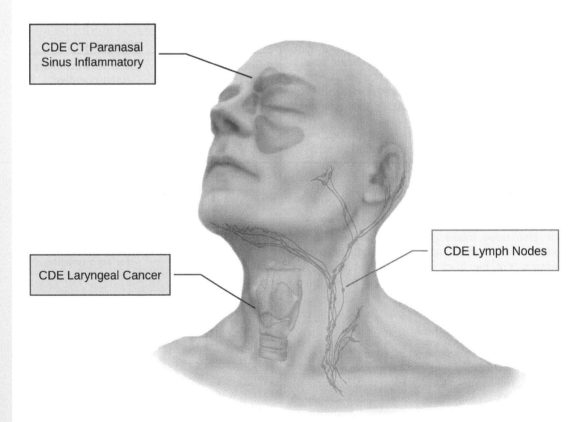

Fig. 4. CDEs currently made available for public use from the ASNR-ACR-RSNA work group for head and neck radiology reporting.

Both formats are also potentially suitable for integration with clinical decision support systems, critical result reporting, and systematic follow-up recommendations.[25]

COMMON DATA ELEMENTS VERSUS STRUCTURED REPORTING: DIFFERENCES

Structured reports standardize the categories or areas for which all radiologists using the given template should describe findings on a particular type of examination, but they do not necessarily ask a specific question or address a key concept related to the underlying disorder and clinical indication of the study. A single CDE is not typically comprehensive enough to represent all of the findings on an examination, and, in contrast, a structured report may force commentary on headings that are superfluous to the case. In addition, unlike CDEs, structured reports do not always have restricted answers for each of the various headings. Although both are better than narrative reporting for use with computers and deep learning systems, the content of CDEs may have advantages in specificity compared with structured reports (Table 1).

THE ROLE OF COMMON DATA ELEMENTS

A CDE is a compromise between those who prefer prose narrative reporting and others who prefer the categorized structured reporting format or the more disease-specific contextual report. A CDE can be inserted into either style of report, leaving individual radiologists with the freedom to choose the format that suits them best but also to take advantage of the benefits of CDEs. Because of this modular concept, multiple CDEs

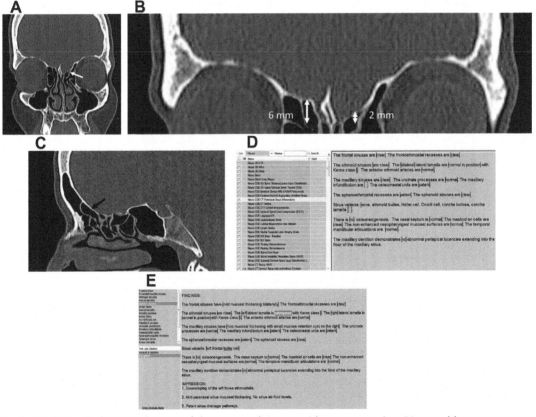

Fig. 5. (A) Coronal reformatted image of the paranasal sinuses without contrast in a 54-year-old woman presenting for otolaryngology evaluation of chronic sinusitis shows asymmetry in the anterior skull base with the left fovea ethmoidalis more inferiorly located (*white arrow*) than the right. (B) Formal measurement of the olfactory fossa depth shows a Keros class II on the right and Keros class I on the left. (C) Also seen on the sagittal reformatted image is an anatomic variant frontal bullar cell (*black arrow*), or posterior frontal recess air cell projecting above the frontal sinus ostium. (D) The head and neck radiologist can insert the CDE for paranasal sinus findings and (E) address each of the key concepts within the CDE with specific answer choices prompted through the CDE template to include the key findings of the anterior skull base anatomy.

could be integrated into a report, as necessary. CDEs may also be inherently built into contextual report templates. As CDEs change and evolve in the future, they can be updated independent of the overall report template a radiologist chooses.

COMMON DATA ELEMENTS VERSUS CONTEXTUAL REPORTING

CDEs perhaps share the most in common with a variant of structured reports called contextual reports. Contextual reporting is based on insertion

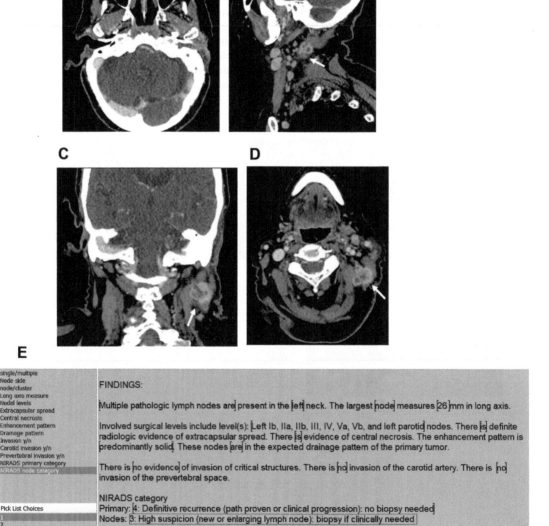

Fig. 6. An 88-year-old woman presented for repeat staging CT of the neck with contrast following subtotal resection of a skin cancer arising from the left pinna with positive surgical margins. (*A*) Axial CT with contrast shows absence of the left pinna with the primary tumor filling the left external auditory canal. (*B*) Numerous pathologic lymph nodes were present in the left neck with (*C, D*) 1 left level IIA lymph node showing areas of internal necrosis with indistinct and spiculated margins concerning for extracapsular spread (*white arrows*). (*E*) CDE implementation in this case prompts the radiologist to provide discrete answers describing these key findings as well as assign NI-RADS categories for both the primary lesion and lymph nodes.

of disease-specific structured reports depending on the imaging protocol, clinical history, or the presence of a finding. For example, in a contextual report for preoperative CT of the sinuses proposed by Mamlouk and colleagues,[40] there are headings to prompt commentary on sinus anatomic variants that otolaryngologists would want to know. Examples of these variants include carotid canal dehiscence, sphenoid sinus septum attachment to the carotid canal, and Onodi cells.[40] Similar to CDEs, the appropriate clinical prompts and pertinent

negatives are included, which guide the radiologist to comment on each appropriate aspect. For both CDE and contextual reports, recognition of the need or context to insert the appropriate template is incumbent on the radiologist, but this could be something that artificial intelligence may automatically trigger in the future.[13] Potential limitations of contextual reports include the radiologist's lack of awareness to insert the appropriate contextual report template or situations in which more than 1 template may be applicable.[25] CDEs may also

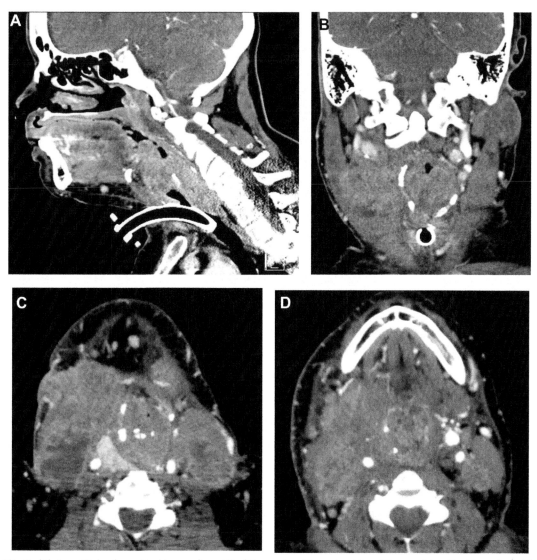

Fig. 7. (A) A sagittal reformatted image from CT of the neck with contrast in a 56-year-old patient transferred for progressive stridor reveals a large glottic to supraglottic mass replacing the epiglottis and narrowing the airway. (B) The tumor has grown laterally beyond the laryngeal skeleton with development of large bilateral lymph nodes. (C) Destructive and invasive changes are seen the thyroid, arytenoid, and cricoid cartilage. (D) Tumor has also grown back to encircle the right internal carotid artery. (E) The key information to provide TNM staging and help organize the report in this complex tumor is prompted through insertion of the CDE. (F) In this situation, the head and neck radiologist may also insert the CDE lymph node, creating the report in a modular fashion.

E

Larynx AP mm measurement	FINDINGS:
Larynx RL mm measurement	
Larynx CC mm measurement	There is a mass in the larynx which measures [38] mm AP by [54] mm RL by [86] mm CC. The mass
Larynx mass center	center is [supraglottic] with glottic and subglottic involvement. The mass shows [enhancement]. The
Larynx mass enhancement	
larynx mass midline extension	mass [does] extend across the midline and it mass [does] narrow the airway. The vocal cord is
larynx mass airway narrowing	[immobile]. There [is no] prevertebral invasion and there [is right] carotid space invasion.
laryngeal mass - cord mobility	
laryngeal mass - prevert invasion	
laryngeal mass - carotid space invasio	There [is] cricoid, arytenoid, and thyroid cartilage invasion. There [is] extension outside the laryngeal
laryngeal mass - cartilage invasion	skeleton.
laryngeal mass - extension beyond sk	
Impression	
	IMPRESSION:

F

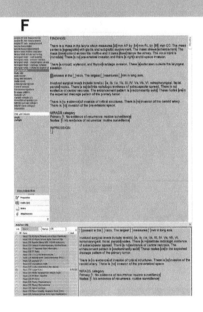

Fig. 7. (continued)

suffer from this first limitation but have more potential to work around the second.

APPLICATIONS OF COMMON DATA ELEMENTS TO THE HEAD AND NECK

Three major radiology societies, the American Society of Neuroradiology (ASNR), the American College of Radiology (ACR), and the RSNA came together to form the Common Data Elements Neuroradiology Workgroup.[3] With the goal of creating CDEs that were clinically relevant, reflected current literature, and tailored for critical decision, the group made a set of CDEs available to the public in 2018. The templates could be implemented into neuroradiology reports and include several CDEs geared for reporting examinations pertinent to imaging of the head and neck. This multisociety collaboration is in keeping with a push from the National Institutes of Health to incorporate CDEs into medical practice and

research.[41] Before this, in August of 2016, the ACR had introduced the Neck Imaging Reporting and Data Systems (NI-RADS) in order to aid consistency in risk stratification and appropriate linked management recommendations for patients with treated head and neck cancer.[42] Although not necessarily labeled as such, the NI-RAD score constituted a significant CDE for head and neck imaging. Since that time, the ASNR-ACR-RSNA workgroup has formally introduced 3 additional head and neck–related CDEs, covering reporting on the paranasal sinuses (inflammatory), cervical lymph nodes, and laryngeal cancer (**Fig. 4**).

COMMON DATA ELEMENT PARANASAL SINUS INFLAMMATORY

The CDE for the paranasal sinus, put forth by the ASNR-ACR-RSNA workgroup, shows elements of a comprehensive structural or contextual report with an emphasis on describing findings for best practice to maximize clinical impact. This CDE broadly covers all of the areas radiologists would review on CT sinus, using a checklist approach for each of the sinuses, their respective drainage pathways, the ostiomeatal units, mastoid air cells, nasopharynx, and maxillary dentition, among other areas (Fig. 5). There is a heading dedicated to description of sinus variants, as well as specific callouts for the anterior skull base in order to describe the position of the lateral lamellae and the Keros classification to assist radiologists' surgical colleagues.[43–45]

COMMON DATA ELEMENT LYMPH NODE

The lymph node CDE from the ASNR-ACR-RSNA workgroup is more modular and can be inserted into multiple examination reports in the head and neck, ranging from MR imaging neck to CT maxillofacial, depending on the need or lymph node findings seen. It could even be inserted into a CT cervical spine or CT angiogram of the neck report. This type of CDE shows the versatility and ability to customize reports to further add clinical value.

This CDE focuses on key lymph node characteristics from size, number, and location to descriptive features, such as central necrosis and signs of extracapsular spread, which are key for differential diagnosis and prognosis (Fig. 6).[46] The lymph node CDE also incorporates the NI-RADS system for both the lymph nodes in question or any primary lesion, if applicable, thus providing a systematic follow-up management plan.[1]

COMMON DATA ELEMENT LARYNGEAL CANCER

The CDE for laryngeal cancer is the most clinically specific of the CDEs and is intended for CT or MR imaging neck but could also be used if a laryngeal cancer is identified incidentally on another type of examination. The laryngeal cancer CDE emphasizes the features necessary to provide the tumor staging (as a component of the TNM classification), which would be valuable to any of the involved providers or the members of a multidisciplinary team to facilitate treatment decision making and follow-up (Fig. 7).[5,6] In its current version, the CDE does not formally state the TNM stage explicitly within the report because there is mixed opinion in the head and neck community as to whether radiologists should report this or leave it for their clinical colleagues to determine.[47] In reports where the laryngeal cancer CDE is activated, it may be appropriate that the lymph node CDE is also used.

SUMMARY

As of early 2020, the ASNR-ACR-RSNA workgroup only has these 3 CDEs for head and neck imaging, along with a CDE for thyroid ultrasonography, leaving an important opportunity for creation of additional CDEs. New CDEs for the temporal bone, nasopharynx, oropharynx, hypopharynx, salivary glands, and deep spaces of the neck, among others, are likely forthcoming. The existing CDEs are also likely to be edited and modified to incorporate future literature-based guidelines and corresponding treatment/follow-up recommendations. The authors speculate that the CDEs will become more specific and modular to allow flexible incorporation into more users' reports and encourage overall use among more individuals and radiology groups to help with future data collection. The CDEs or CDE concepts may also be incorporated into contextual reports, which the authors also expect to gain traction compared with standard structured reporting.

With future advances to natural language processing and deep learning convolutional neural networks, real-time computer understanding of the radiologist's words is likely to continue to improve.[48] This may one day allow automated or suggested insertion of CDEs into a report. Completely computer-generated CDE creation may also become possible as artificial image interpretation improves.

Adoption of CDEs into the current practice of head and neck radiologists will be essential to help drive these future possibilities. Groups that embrace CDEs now will be instrumental in helping to influence the direction and future content of CDEs, particularly in the head and neck realm, where imaging plays such a critical role in diagnosis, staging, surgical planning, therapy selection, and monitoring of disease response.

ACKNOWLEDGMENTS

The authors thank Caroline O'Driscoll, MS (USC Mark and Mary Stevens Neuroimaging and Informatics Institute, University of Southern California, Keck School of Medicine, Los Angeles, CA) for the artwork in Fig. 4.

DISCLOSURE

The authors have nothing to disclose.

REFERENCES

1. Aiken AH, Rath TJ, Anzai Y, et al. ACR neck imaging reporting and data systems (NI-RADS): a white

paper of the ACR NI-RADS Committee. J Am Coll Radiol 2018;15:1097–108.

2. Rubin DL, Kahn CE. Common data elements in radiology. Radiology 2017;283:837–44.

3. Flanders AE, Jordan JE. The ASNR-ACR-RSNA common data elements project: what will it do for the house of neuroradiology? AJNR Am J Neuroradiol 2019;40:14–8.

4. Winget MD, Baron JA, Spitz MR, et al. Development of common data elements: the experience of and recommendations from the early detection research network. Int J Med Inform 2003;70:41–8.

5. Glastonbury CM, Mukherji SK, O'Sullivan B, et al. Setting the Stage for 2018: How the changes in the american joint committee on cancer/union for international cancer control. AJNR Am J Neuroradiol 2017;38:2231–7.

6. Lydiatt WM, Patel SG, O'Sullivan B, et al. Head and Neck cancers-major changes in the American Joint Committee on cancer eighth edition cancer staging manual. CA Cancer J Clin 2017;67:122–37.

7. Bates DW, Gawande AA. Improving safety with information technology. N Engl J Med 2003;348: 2526–34.

8. Herold CJ, Lewin JS, Wibmer AG, et al. Imaging in the Age of Precision Medicine: Summary of the Proceedings of the 10th Biannual Symposium of the International Society for Strategic Studies in Radiology. Radiology 2016;279:226–38.

9. Warzel DB, Andonaydis C, McCurry B, et al. Common data element (CDE) management and deployment in clinical trials. AMIA Annu Symp Proc 2003; 2003:1048.

10. Haacke EM, Duhaime AC, Gean AD, et al. Common data elements in radiologic imaging of traumatic brain injury. J Magn Reson Imaging 2010;32: 516–43.

11. Loring DW, Lowenstein DH, Barbaro NM, et al. Common data elements in epilepsy research: development and implementation of the NINDS epilepsy CDE project. Epilepsia 2011;52:1186–91.

12. Rosenkrantz AB, Nicola GN, Allen B, et al. MACRA, MIPS, and the new medicare quality payment program: an update for radiologists. J Am Coll Radiol 2017;14:316–23.

13. Kohli M, Alkasab T, Wang K, et al. Bending the artificial intelligence curve for radiology: informatics tools from ACR and RSNA. J Am Coll Radiol 2019; 16:1464–70.

14. Khorasani R. Clinical decision support in radiology: what is it, why do we need it, and what key features make it effective? J Am Coll Radiol 2006;3:142–3.

15. Boland GW, Thrall JH, Gazelle GS, et al. Decision support for radiologist report recommendations. J Am Coll Radiol 2011;8:819–23.

16. Chen JY, Sippel Schmidt TM, Carr CD, et al. Enabling the next-generation radiology report:

17. Ganeshan D, Duong PT, Probyn L, et al. Structured reporting in radiology. Acad Radiol 2018;25:66–73.

18. Srinivasa Babu A, Brooks ML. The malpractice liability of radiology reports: minimizing the risk. Radiographics 2015;35:547–54.

19. Cannavale A, Santoni M, Mancarella P, et al. Malpractice in radiology: what should you worry about? Radiol Res Pract 2013;2013:219259.

20. Henshaw D, Okawa G, Ching K, et al. Access to Radiology Reports via an Online Patient Portal: Experiences of Referring Physicians and Patients. J Am Coll Radiol 2015;12:582–6.e1.

21. Okawa G, Ching K, Qian H, et al. Automatic release of radiology reports via an online patient portal. J Am Coll Radiol 2017;14:1219–21.

22. Cai T, Giannopoulos AA, Yu S, et al. Natural language processing technologies in radiology research and clinical applications. Radiographics 2016;36:176–91.

23. Wallis A, McCoubrie P. The radiology report–are we getting the message across? Clin Radiol 2011;66: 1015–22.

24. Hickey P. Standardization of Roentgen-ray Reports. American Journal of Roentgenology 1922;9:422-5.

25. Shea LAG, Towbin AJ. The state of structured reporting: the nuance of standardized language. Pediatr Radiol 2019;49:500–8.

26. Kahn CE, Heilbrun ME, Applegate KE. From guidelines to practice: how reporting templates promote the use of radiology practice guidelines. J Am Coll Radiol 2013;10:268–73.

27. Radiological Society of North America. RadReport template library; 2020. Available at: www.radreport. org. Accessed April 30, 2020.

28. Langlotz CP, Caldwell SA. The completeness of existing lexicons for representing radiology report information. J Digit Imaging 2002;15(Suppl 1): 201–5.

29. Rubin DL. Creating and curating a terminology for radiology: ontology modeling and analysis. J Digit Imaging 2008;21:355–62.

30. Langlotz CP. RadLex: a new method for indexing on-line educational materials. Radiographics 2006;26: 1595–7.

31. Lin E, Powell DK, Kagetsu NJ. Efficacy of a checklist-style structured radiology reporting template in reducing resident misses on cervical spine computed tomography examinations. J Digit Imaging 2014;27:588–93.

32. Rocha DM, Brasil LM, Lamas JM, et al. Evidence of the benefits, advantages and potentialities of the structured radiological report: An integrative review. Artif Intell Med 2020;102:101770.

33. Chung CY, Makeeva V, Yan J, et al. Improving billing accuracy through enterprise-wide standardized

structured reporting with cross-divisional shared templates. J Am Coll Radiol 2020;17:157–64.

34. Larson DB, Towbin AJ, Pryor RM, et al. Improving consistency in radiology reporting through the use of department-wide standardized structured reporting. Radiology 2013;267:240–50.

35. Cabana MD, Rand CS, Powe NR, et al. Why don't physicians follow clinical practice guidelines? A framework for improvement. JAMA 1999;282: 1458–65.

36. Gunderman RB, McNeive LR. Is structured reporting the answer? Radiology 2014;273:7–9.

37. Weiss DL, Langlotz CP. Structured reporting: patient care enhancement or productivity nightmare? Radiology 2008;249:739–47.

38. Ritzer Ross J. Structured reporting: resistance is futile. Radiology Business2019.

39. Johnson AJ, Chen MY, Swan JS, et al. Cohort study of structured reporting compared with conventional dictation. Radiology 2009;253:74–80.

40. Mamlouk MD, Chang PC, Saket RR. Contextual radiology reporting: a new approach to neuroradiology structured templates. AJNR Am J Neuroradiol 2018;39:1406–14.

41. Rubinstein YR, McInnes P. NIH/NCATS/GRDR® Common Data Elements: A leading force for standardized data collection. Contemp Clin Trials 2015; 42:78–80.

42. Aiken AH, Farley A, Baugnon KL, et al. Implementation of a novel surveillance template for head and neck cancer: neck imaging reporting and data system (NI-RADS). J Am Coll Radiol 2016;13:743–6.e1.

43. Bayrak S, Aktuna Belgin C, Orhan K. Evaluation of the relationship between olfactory fossa measurements and nasal septum deviation for endoscopic sinus surgery. J Craniofac Surg 2020;31(3): 801–3.

44. Huang BY, Lloyd KM, DelGaudio JM, et al. Failed endoscopic sinus surgery: spectrum of CT findings in the frontal recess. Radiographics 2009;29: 177–95.

45. O'Brien WT, Hamelin S, Weitzel EK. The preoperative sinus CT: avoiding a "CLOSE" call with surgical complications. Radiology 2016;281:10–21.

46. Wreesmann VB, Katabi N, Palmer FL, et al. Influence of extracapsular nodal spread extent on prognosis of oral squamous cell carcinoma. Head Neck 2016;38(Suppl 1):E1192–9.

47. Ko B, Parvathaneni U, Hudgins PA, et al. Do radiologists report the TNM staging in radiology reports for head and neck cancers? a national survey study. AJNR Am J Neuroradiol 2016;37:1504–9.

48. Chen MC, Ball RL, Yang L, et al. Deep learning to classify radiology free-text reports. Radiology 2018;286:845–52.

Moving?

Make sure your subscription moves with you!

To notify us of your new address, find your **Clinics Account Number** (located on your mailing label above your name), and contact customer service at:

Email: journalscustomerservice-usa@elsevier.com

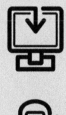

800-654-2452 (subscribers in the U.S. & Canada)
314-447-8871 (subscribers outside of the U.S. & Canada)

Fax number: 314-447-8029

**Elsevier Health Sciences Division
Subscription Customer Service
3251 Riverport Lane
Maryland Heights, MO 63043**

*To ensure uninterrupted delivery of your subscription, please notify us at least 4 weeks in advance of move.

Printed and bound by CPI Group (UK) Ltd, Croydon, CR0 4YY

03/10/2024

01040371-0011